Spas for Your Home

Spas for Your Home

Cristina Paredes Benítez

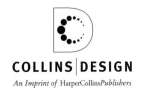

COLLINS | DESIGN

An Imprint of HarperCollins*Publishers*

SPAS FOR YOUR HOME
Copyright © 2005 by Collins DESIGN and LOFT Publications

HarperCollins books may be purchased for educational, business, or sales promotional use.
For information, please write: Special Markets Department, HarperCollins Publishers Inc.,
10 East 53rd Street, New York, NY 10022

First Edition

First published in 2005 by:
Collins Design
An Imprint of HarperCollinsPublishers
10 East 53rd Street
New York, NY 10022
Tel.: (212) 207-7000
Fax: (212) 207-7654
HarperDesign@harpercollins.com
www.harpercollins.com

Distributed throughout the world by:
HarperCollinsPublishers
10 East 53rd Street
New York, NY 10022
Fax: (212) 207-7654

Packager by
LOFT Publications
Via Laietana 32, 4° Of. 92
08003 Barcelona, Spain
Tel.: +34 932 688 088
Fax: +34 932 687 073
loft@loftpublications.com
www.loftpublications.com

Editor:
Cristina Paredes Benítez

Art Director:
Mireia Casanovas Soley

Layout:
Ignasi Gracia Blanco

Library of Congress Cataloging-in-Publication Data

Paredes Benítez, Cristina.
  Spas for your home / Cristina Paredes Benítez.-- 1st ed.
    p. cm.
  ISBN 0-06-074978-4 (hardcover)
  1. Bathrooms. 2. Spa pools. 3. Sauna. 4. Interior decoration. I. Title.
  NK2117.B33P37 2005
  747.7'8--dc22
                                    2005021770

Printed by: Anman Gràfiques del Vallès
Spain

D.L: B-35.967-05

First Printing, 2005

Summary

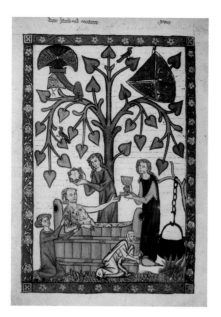

Originally, a spa was a place with curative waters, such as mineral and thermal waters. Taking these baths was part of caring for one's health and one's body in various cultures over the course of centuries. We find many examples in history: from the Egyptian purification rituals to the Roman baths to the pre-Columbian steam baths, or *temazcalli*. Today we can say that the concept of the spa has been not just retained, but extended and expanded with the addition of other therapies that also contribute to our well-being and a healthy lifestyle. The spa is more popular now than ever, and the trend continues as it becomes more affordable. The opportunity to enjoy spa therapies on a regular basis is within the reach of many more people, and the ability to have a spa in one's own home is now a reality. Increasing numbers of people are considering the possibility of a home spa, expanding the swimming pool and terrace areas or including hydromassage baths and showers in their bathrooms.

Water has many applications: therapies for rheumatism and rehabilitation, weight loss, fitness, and just relaxing after a long day at work. Thanks to technological advances and new materials, we now have more comfortable saunas, bathrooms, and spas with many more features. The new materials (porcelains and resins) have supplemented the traditional materials, such as wood, marble, and ceramics, so we can create spaces that are functional and have character. Traditionally, the indispensable elements of a spa have been saunas, steam baths, and Jacuzzis, although a hydromassage column in the shower can produce the same effect of being either relaxing or invigorating. In the spa culture, it's not just the technology of bathtubs and showers that plays an important role. It is also essential to create an appropriate, harmonious setting in which to enjoy a relaxing session. Either in the bathroom or in other rooms designed especially for this purpose, the setting should help us leave our worries behind and eliminate stress. The rooms must be relaxing; the décor and the materials must be conducive to rest and meditation. The spa in our home should be a true paradise of peace and tranquility.

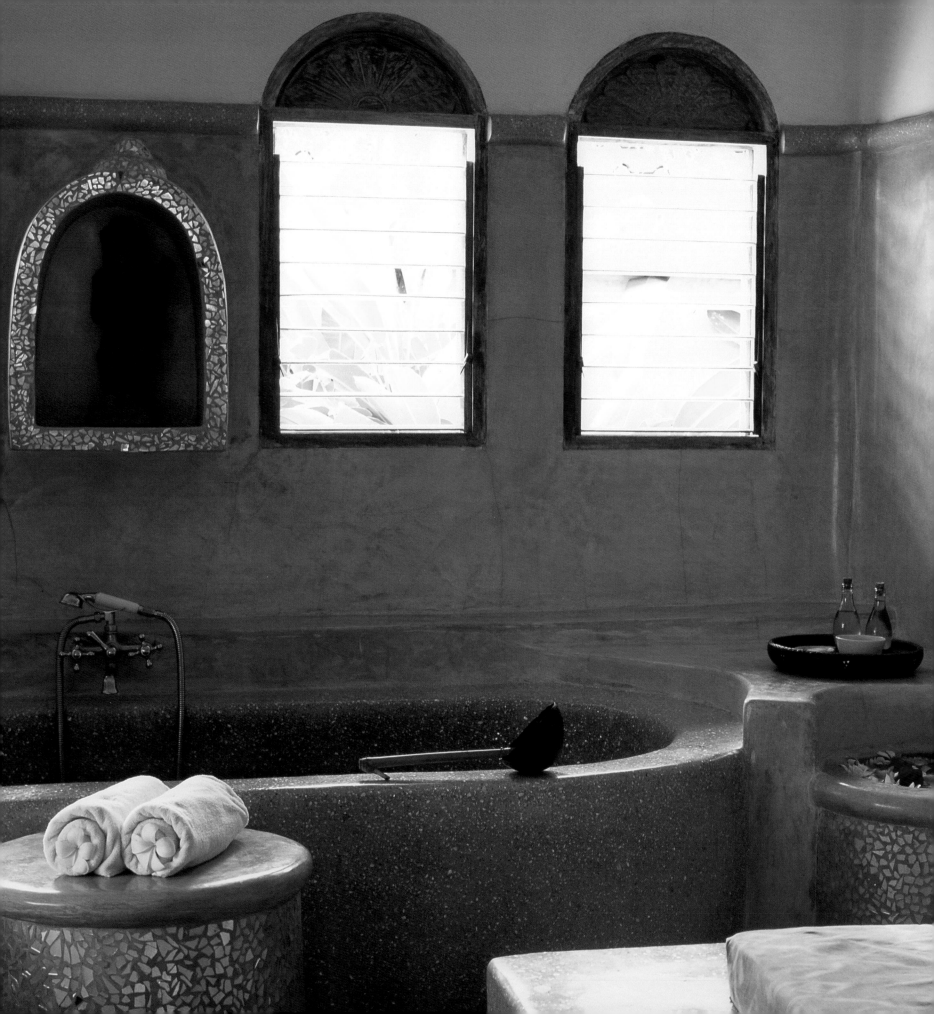

THE HISTORY OF SPAS

The hypotheses regarding the origins of the word *spa* are varied: some have suggested that it derives from the Walloon word *espa*, which means spring, although it may stem from the Latin word *spagere*, or even from an acronym of the phrases *salute per aqua* or *sanitas per aqua*. Other sources point to the name of the Belgian city Spa, which is famous for its thermal springs. In any case, there is no doubt that nowadays the word suggests a concept that quickly brings to mind health, curative therapies, well-being, and relaxation.

The earliest civilizations viewed water as a sacred, as well as curative, element. Furthermore, as many primitive cultures considered illnesses to be divine punishments, water was used for precisely this reason in purification ceremonies. It was the Greeks, however, who were the greatest standard-bearers of the curative properties of water; even their baths were dedicated to different deities, such as Asclepius, the god of medicine. Hippocrates, who lived 400 years before Christ, believed that the secret to good health lay in keeping the body in equilibrium, which one could achieve through water therapy, a proper diet, massages, and stability of mind. Some of the treatments applied then—such as jets of water, steam baths, and mud baths—continue to be used in spas today.

Influenced by the Greeks, the Romans introduced a social parameter to their public baths, which eventually came to serve as meeting places. It is believed that at the peak of the Roman Empire, as many as 370 gallons of water were used in these baths per person per day. In addition to public baths (*balnea publica* or *thermae*), there were also private baths (*balnea privata*) and baths in homes (*balnea*), although only the highest social classes could afford such a luxury. Interestingly, it was the presence of the Roman army that sometimes prompted the construction of baths in Europe—they were used not just to cure injured soldiers, but also as centers of recreation.

After the fall of the Roman Empire and through the Middle Ages, the customs of hygiene and caring for one's body fell out of favor, even in distinguished families. One should, however, point out the remarkable exception of southern Europe, which was occupied by Muslims for eight centuries. Islam held hydrotherapy in high esteem, which—as it required a certain level of personal hygiene of those participating in certain religious ceremonies—gave rise to the culture of bathing in those regions and even saw it turn into a tradition.

From the fifteenth century on, beginning at the height of the Renaissance, hydrotherapy was rediscovered in Europe thanks to a renewed interest in the ancient classics. Doctors and scholars published a number of treatises on the characteristics and effects of medicinal waters.

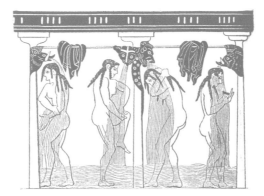

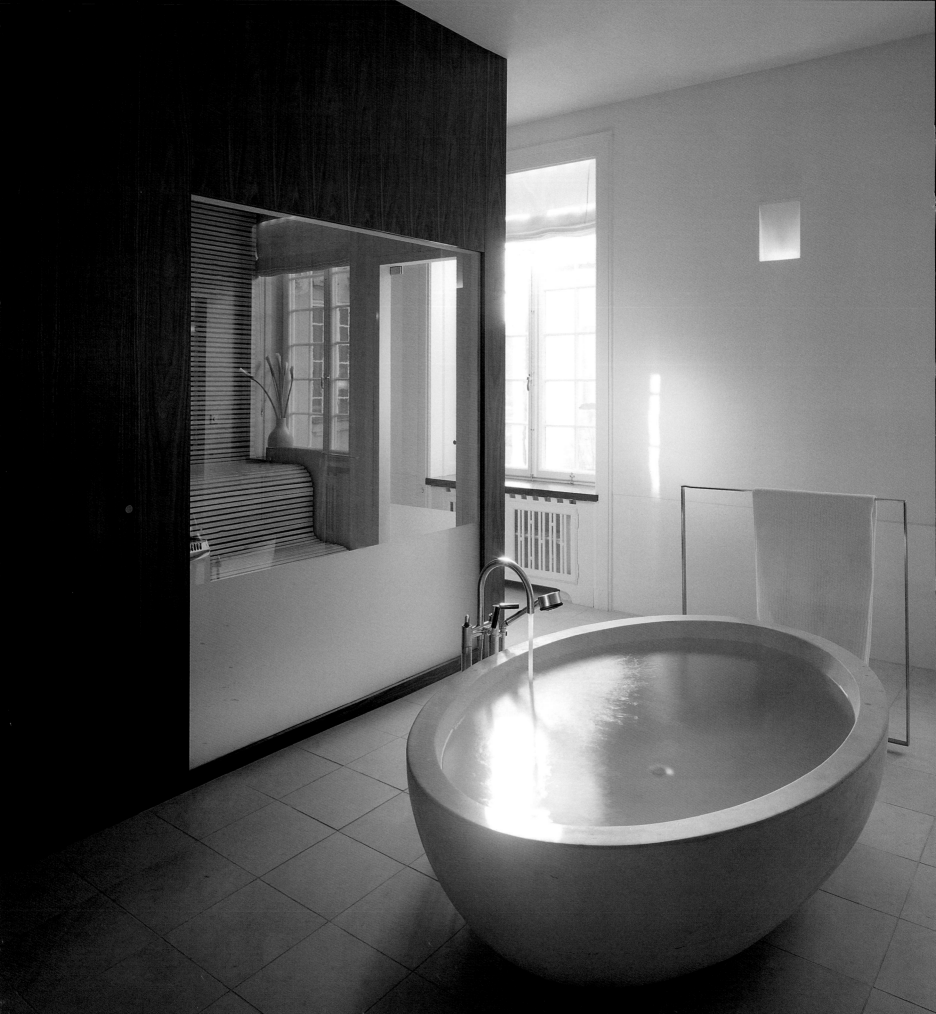

Toward the end of the eighteenth century, the doctors Sigmund and Johann Hahn began to study the applications of hydrotherapy as preventive medicine and as a therapeutic treatment for a range of illnesses. From that point on, spas and water-based treatments spread rapidly. However, society's interest in spas has continued to evolve: while in the nineteenth century, they were thought of as being exclusively curative in purpose, spas are now understood to entail much more—to a degree, the original spirit of the ritual of water has been reborn, and the social dimension of the experience has gained ground as well. One should also point out that the study of the medical benefits of these therapies has also advanced dramatically, and what was once based on faith is now backed up by science. Spas are once again associated with a healthy lifestyle, recreation, and conviviality. Furthermore, their presence has even come to grace our homes; advances in technology allow us to easily install hydromassage baths, steam baths, and saunas at home. Thus, to counteract the hectic pace of modern-day life, we can benefit from hydrotherapy to enhance our overall health and well-being.

HYDROMASSAGE

When the Jacuzzi brothers invented the portable hydrotherapy pump to alleviate their arthritis, a new therapeutic technique was born: hydromassage. Out of all the therapies offered by spas, hydromassage is perhaps the most widely known. It is made up of jets of water that massage the body at varying degrees of pressure and temperatures. The different intensities of water relax the body, reduce stress, activate circulation, and eliminate muscular tension. Hydromassage is associated with a healthy lifestyle as well as with an atmosphere of harmony and relaxation. Hydromassage baths, as well as columns and cabins, offer the body a number of benefits. Their having been perfected over time has culminated in today's integrated systems, which include baths, showers, columns, cabins, pools, and a full range of cubicles to enclose whichever system one chooses. Manufacturers have developed high-quality finishes, a wide range of features, and competitive prices, all of which spell out the perfect combination for every home.

The projects shown in this book also aim to offer well-being accompanied by a carefully planned décor. The wide variety of baths, showers, and cabins on the market can be integrated into bedrooms or, alternatively, installed in the main bathroom. We present a wide range of materials that can be used to convert spas into places for resting and taking care of one's body. Alongside the latest advances in hydrotherapy, we have also focused on the details and complementary features that make them more enjoyable: ergonomic designs, remote controls to regulate water and steam pressure intensity, thermostatic faucets, built-in stereos, slip-proof seats and floors, and even infrared lamps for drying towels.

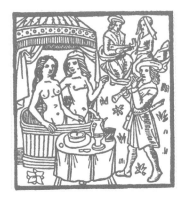

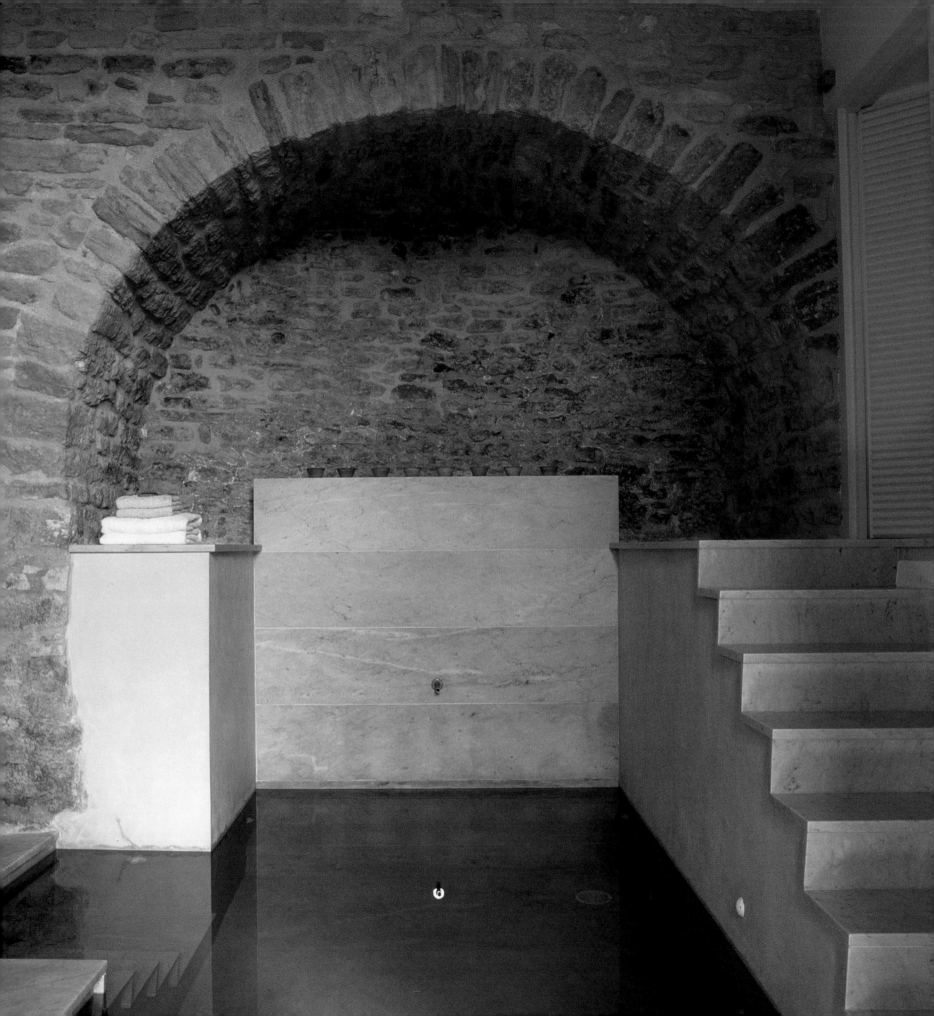

In some cases, these services are located outdoors, or even include swimming pools. As spas engage in dialogue with and blend into the architecture of these houses and terraces, the result is the perfect spot to relax, have fun, or take care of one's body. A spa creates a dynamic space, regardless of whether it is located outdoors or in a purpose-built pavilion. The pools shown in these projects are not, however, excessively large spaces, as they typically serve to complement spa treatments and to enhance their benefits. As an example of this, one can benefit from going from a warm bath to the cold water of a pool to activate the blood flow, or from engaging in aqua-gym, in which one performs exercises in the water.

SAUNA

The sauna is one of the most widespread of spa therapies. Originally from Scandinavia, this system of dry heat is used to clean and detoxify the skin. Additionally, by sweating, one consumes calories, and the heat helps to stabilize blood pressure and to reduce stress. One of the most important components of a sauna is its chamber, in which everything—from walls to benches—is crafted from wood. However, the most essential element in a sauna is its stove, which is used to heat a dish of stones, onto which one casts water to create steam and, in doing so, the atmosphere we traditionally associate with the sauna. The sophisticated systems available today for generating heat also maintain a stable temperature and a homogenous distribution of heat, while newer materials and construction techniques allow for a perfect insulation of the interior and natural ventilation. Some companies have further developed the concept of the hydrosauna, which entails a hydromassage cabin that includes the mechanisms needed for one to enjoy a sauna in the very same space.

It may seem that there is little room for innovation in the design of saunas due to their technical requirements, yet the area of interplay between sauna and home is a fertile field for the imagination, in which one can craft a wide range of highly original and personal spaces. Though each project we examine in this book exhibits a unique aesthetic, what links them all is the way in which they strive to promote well-being and make living a healthy lifestyle possible.

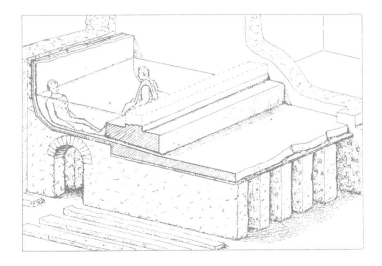

A Spa in Darmstadt

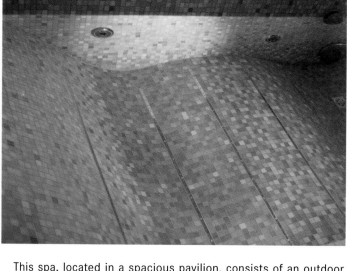

This spa, located in a spacious pavilion, consists of an outdoor sauna, a pool, two showers, and a hydromassage bath. Its footprint is irregular, to adapt to the site, and positions the building next to a garden. The perimeter is enclosed almost entirely by glass walls, which allows for natural light to enter the building as well as for people inside it to enjoy views of the garden. It consists of one open space, except for the showers, which are located in a separate section half hidden by walls clad in tesseras that show the same pattern as in the bath. White and blue are alternated to create a light-filled and calm atmosphere, which is perfect for both swimming and relaxation. At night, a system of embedded lights provides for a warm and serene light that resembles the natural illumination during the day. The uniqueness of this spa is also due to the nature of the system that makes it run: the hot water and electricity are obtained through the use of numerous solar panels, which provide for a clean and renewable source of energy.

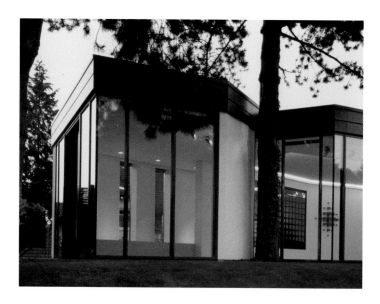

Architect: **Auris Architekten**
Location: **Darmstadt, Germany**
Photos © **Dieter Leistner/Artur**

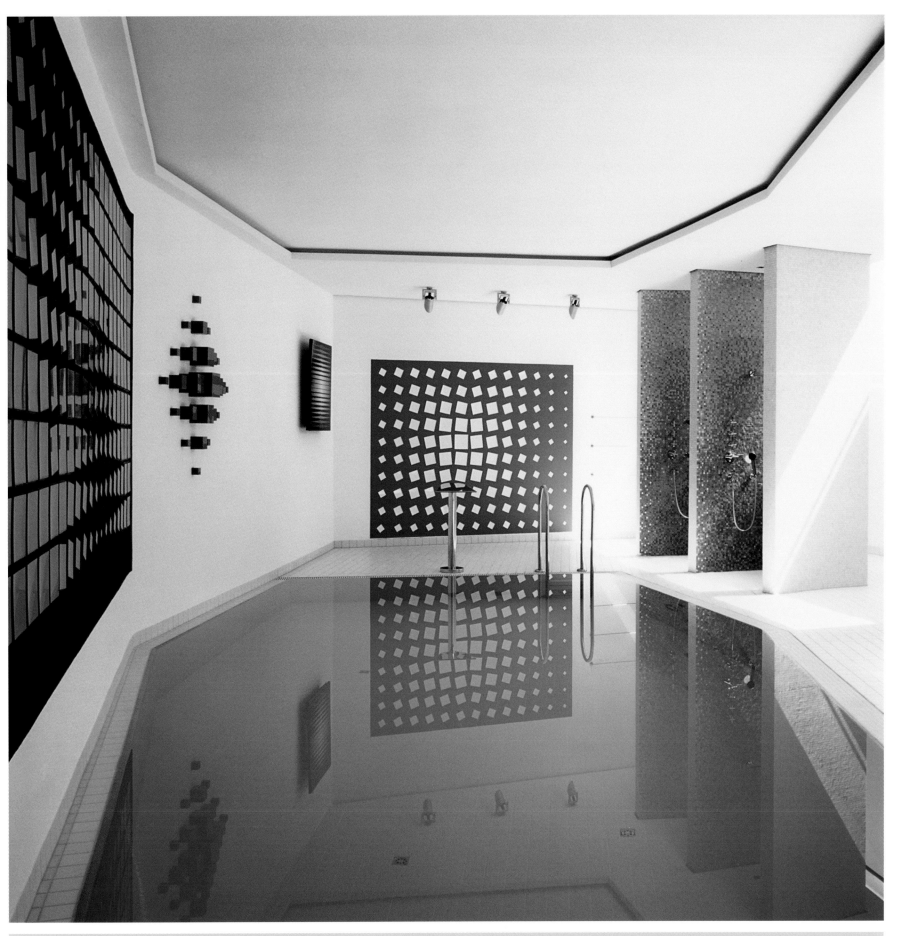

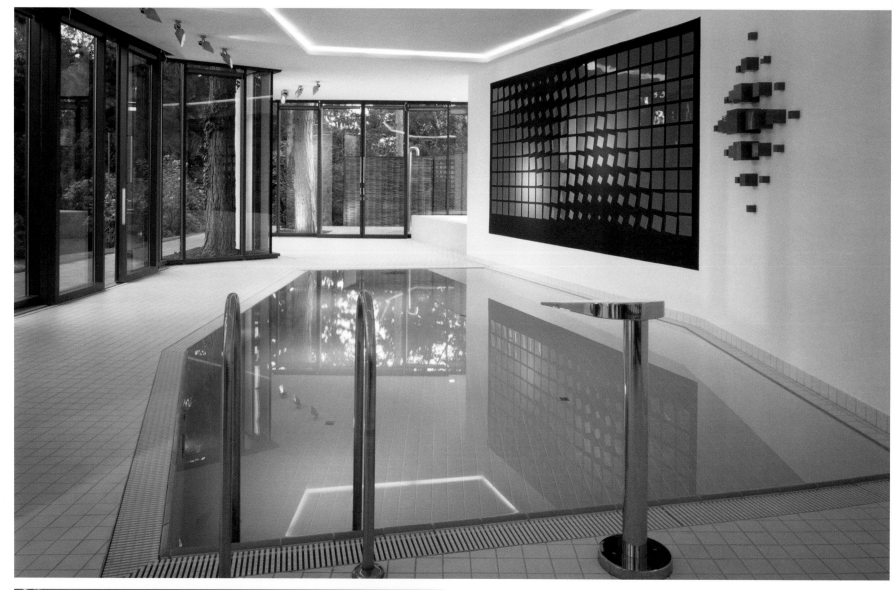

The simple lines of its architecture and its light-filled atmosphere are two of the defining characteristics of this spa.

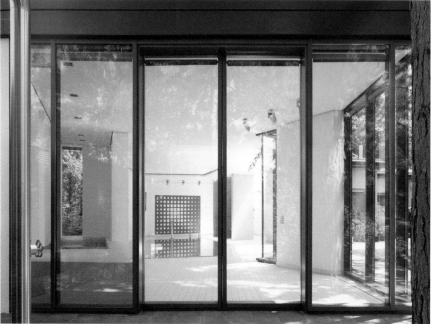

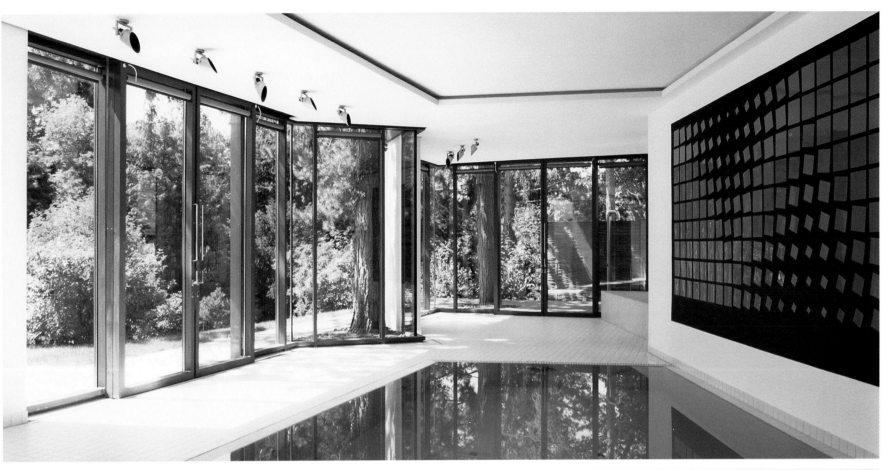

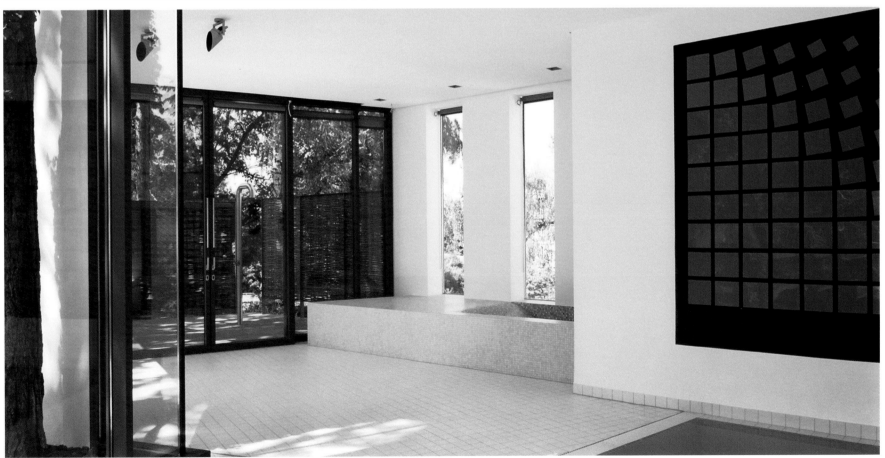

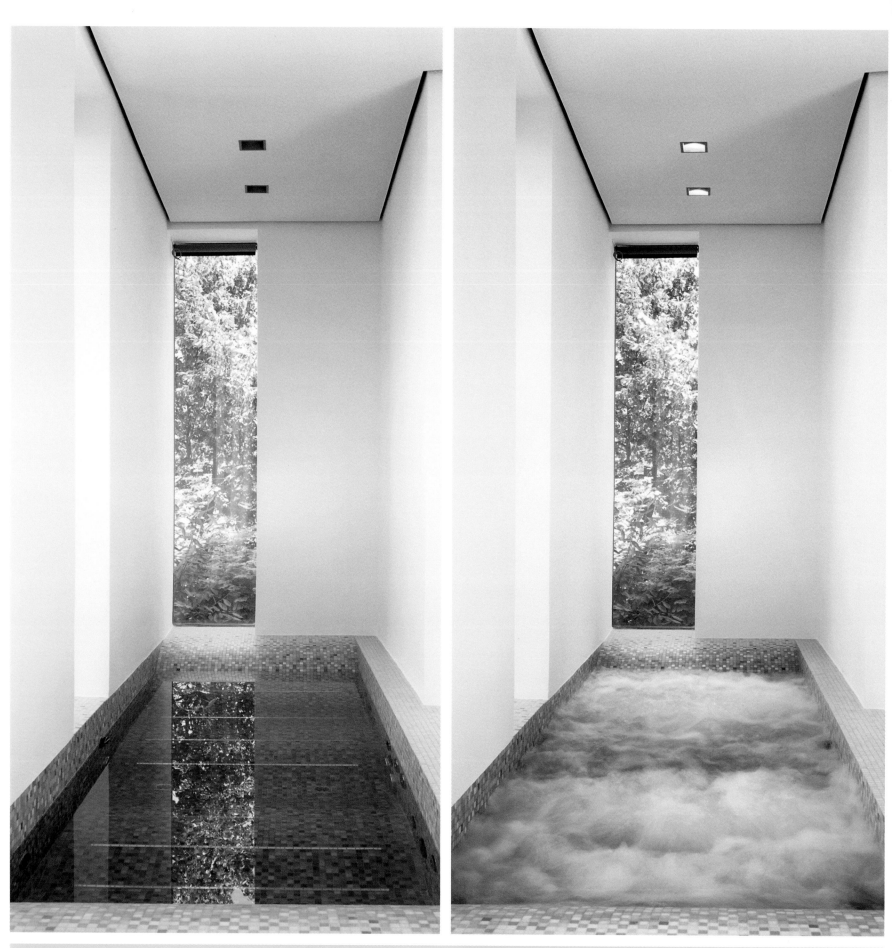

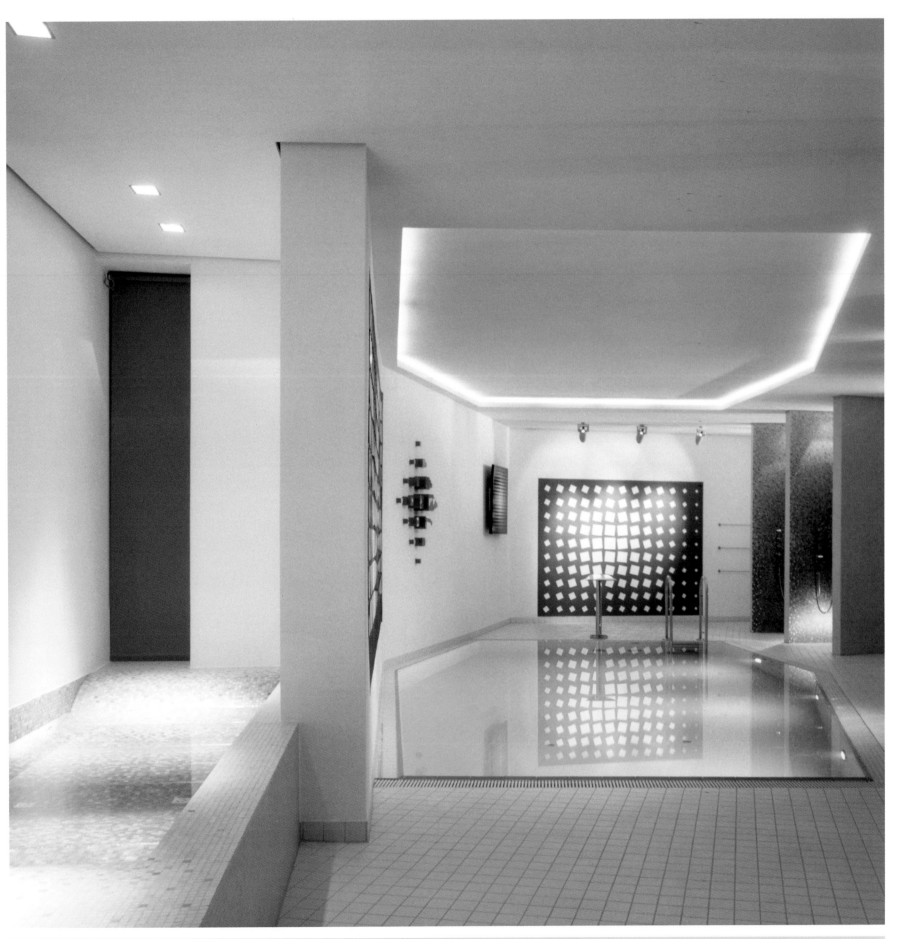

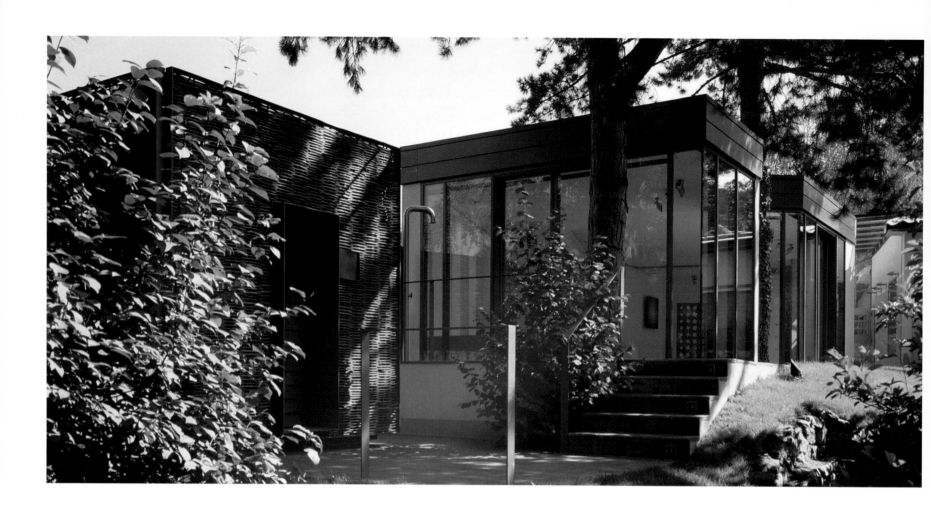

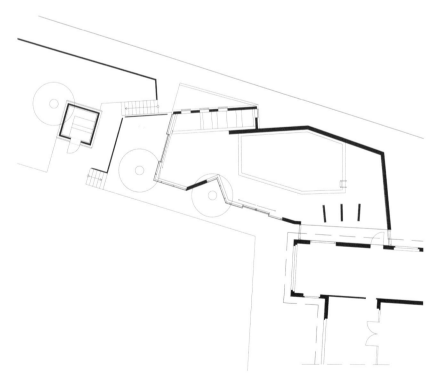

Plan

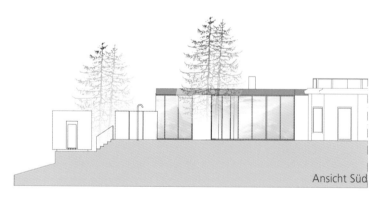

Ansicht Süd

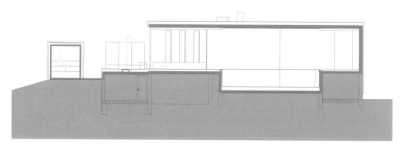

Sections

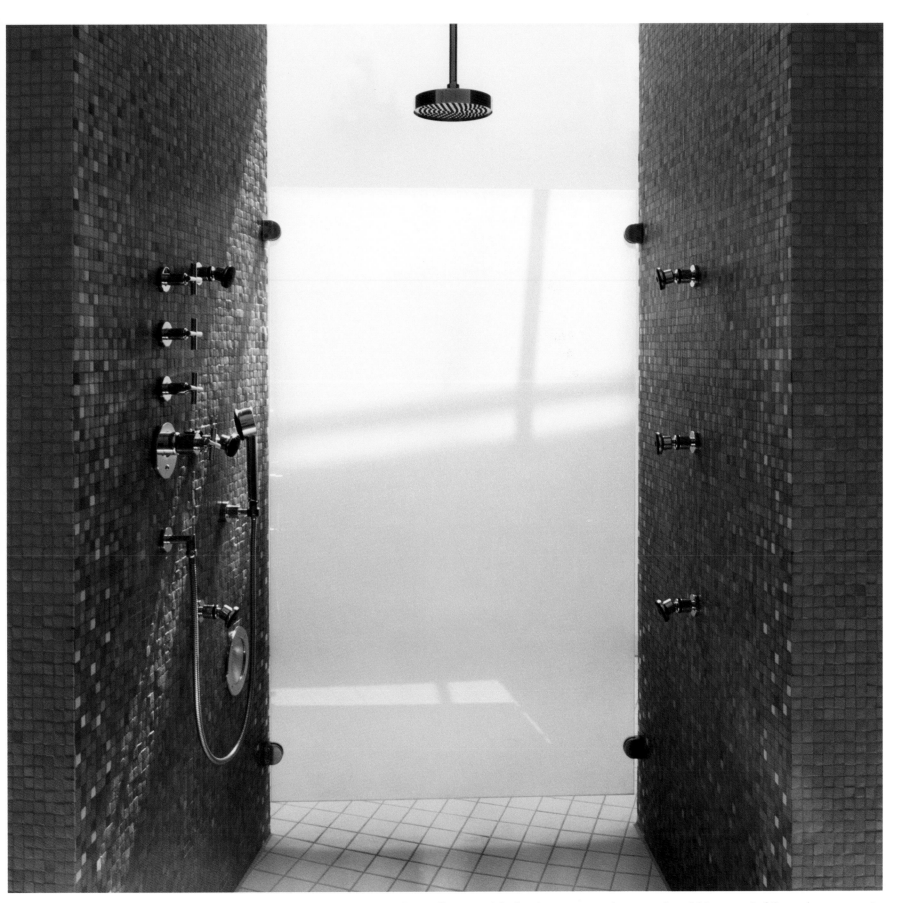

Solar panels generate the hot water for the showers and the pool, as well as part of the heating system, saving as much as thirty percent of the spa's energy costs.

A House
in Aobadai

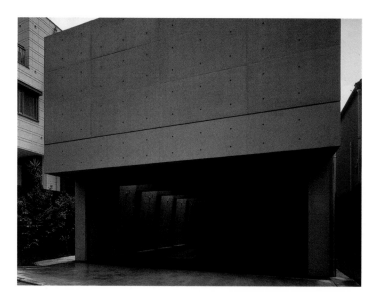

This house is located on Daikanyama Hill, one of the most fashionable neighborhoods in Tokyo. The client, an executive smitten with the world of automobiles, acquired the site with the intention of building his home there, as well as having a place to entertain clients and friends. The first floor is the location of the common family rooms and the area reserved for guests, which includes a terrace with a hydromassage tub. This ample space, situated atop the garage, allows one to bathe in the open air while surrounded in a tranquil and minimalist atmosphere. An artificial, glass-bottomed brook flows slowly alongside one of the walls. This is an atmosphere bathed in an evidently Japanese aesthetic, whose austerity is defined by the materials used—they are left visible to the eye throughout. This spa allows its guests to enjoy serenity and isolation, yet can also serve as the center of a social gathering.

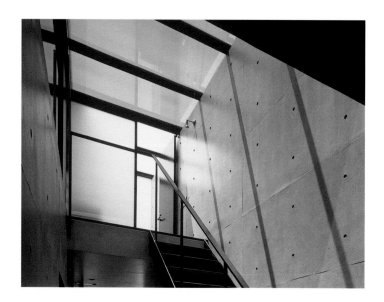

Architect: **Satoshi Okada Architects**
Location: **Tokyo, Japan**
Photos © **Satoshi Okada Architects**

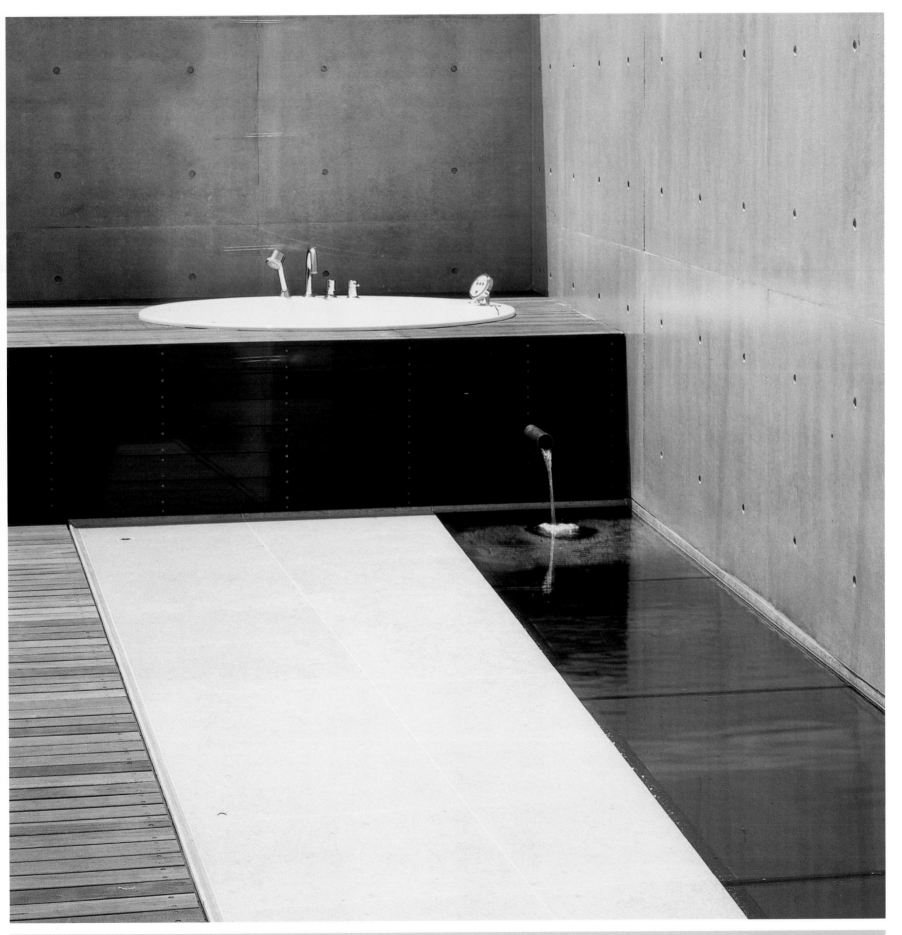

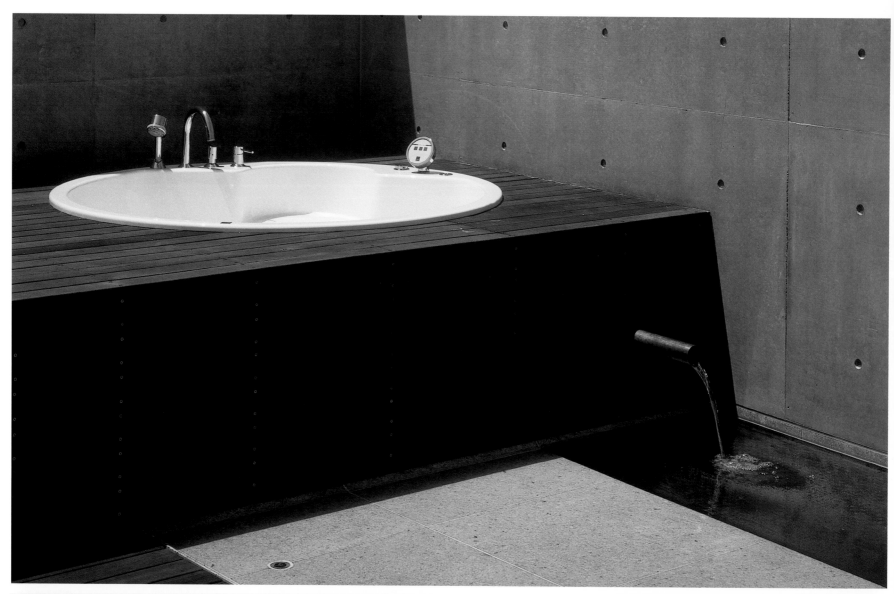

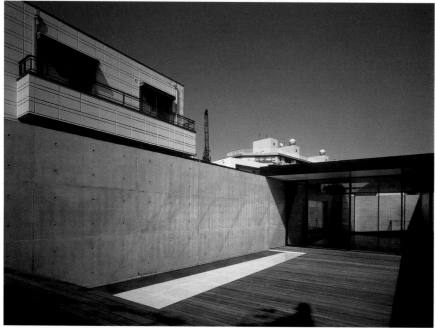

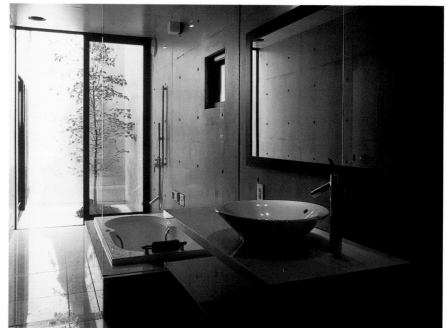

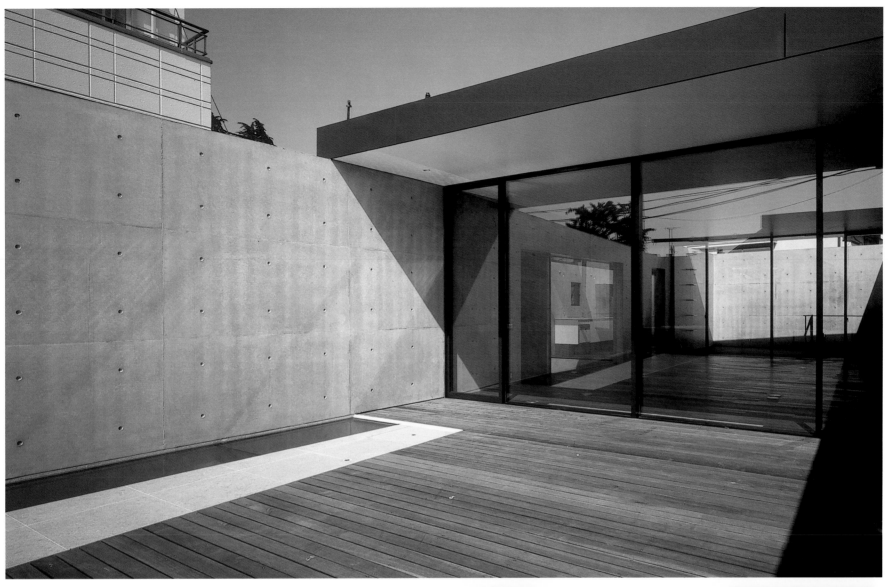

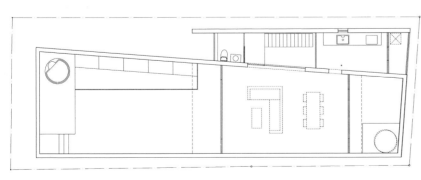

Plan

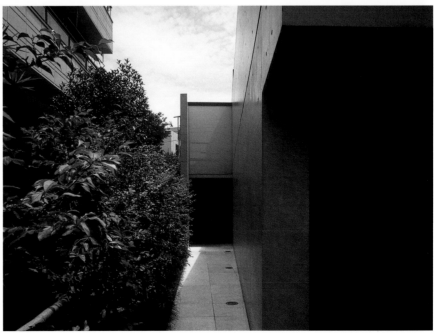

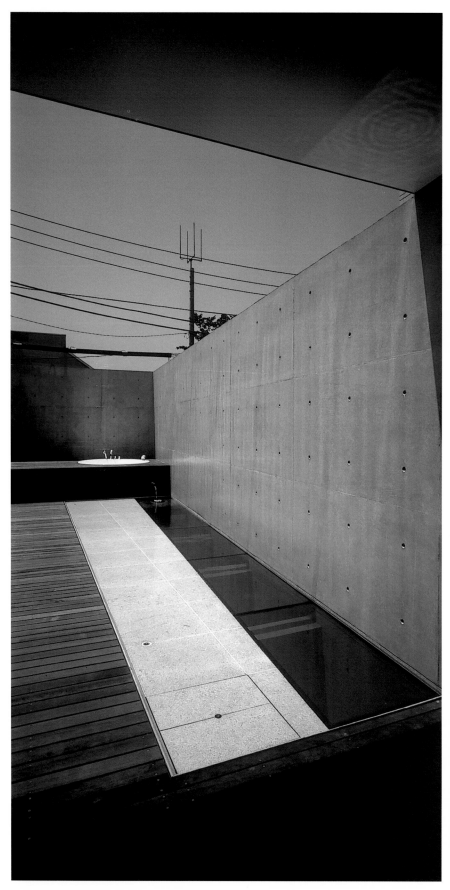

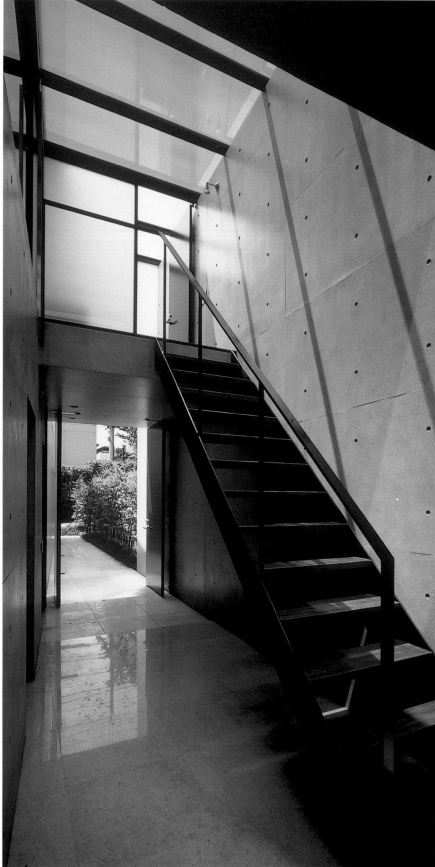

The simplicity of the architecture and the materials used define the spaces of this house and foster an atmosphere that is serene and also thoroughly modern.

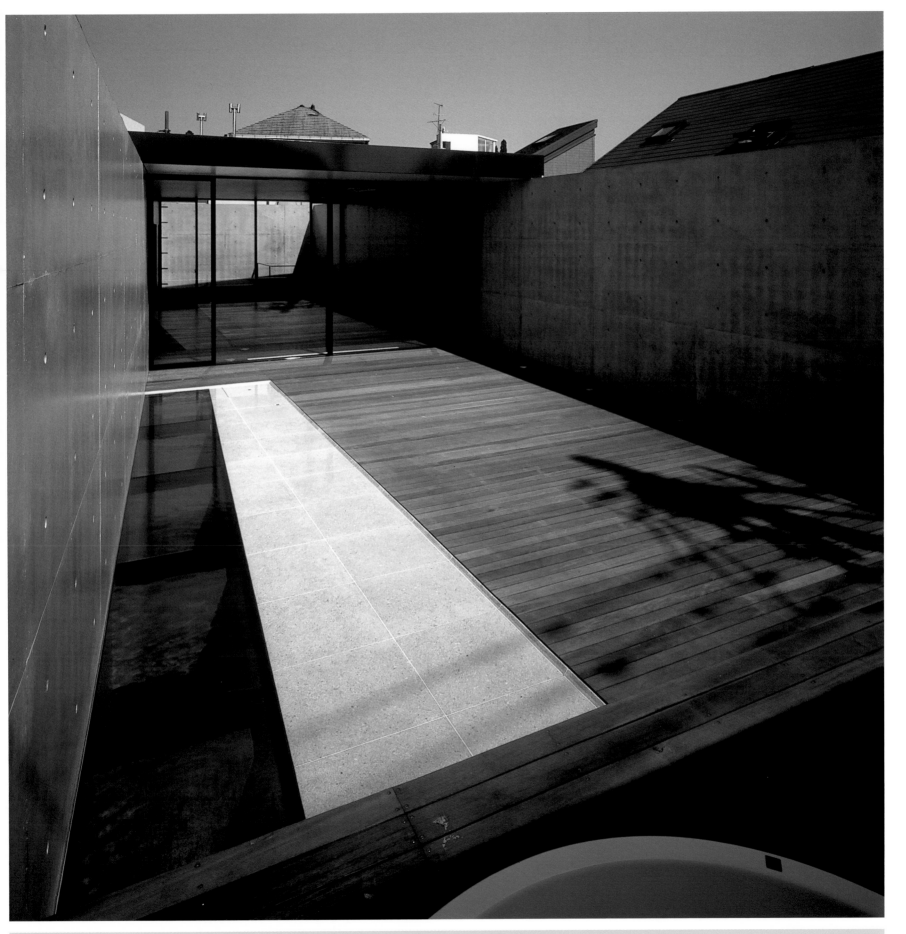

Windmill House

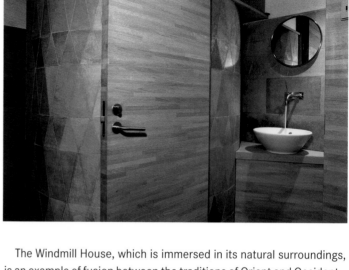

The Windmill House, which is immersed in its natural surroundings, is an example of fusion between the traditions of Orient and Occident—here, one can see the combination of Japanese aesthetics with Scandinavian tradition. Wood and limestone are the principal materials used, and blend into the natural environment to create an organic architecture in keeping with the principles espoused by Frank Lloyd Wright. Traditional Scandinavian customs, such as the sauna and cold- and hot-water baths, are also present in this small house. A hallway finished in wood and stone serves as a dressing room and doubles as an entrance to the bathing area, where the sauna is located. This is one of the most important elements in the house, which—due to its small size—forced the cold-water bath to be placed outside. The garden, in which one can hear a constant flowing of water throughout, is designed in a Japanese style. This magical place makes purification of body and spirit—as well as communion with nature—a real possibility.

Architect: **Wingårdh**
Location: **Malmö, Sweden**
Photos © **James Silverman**

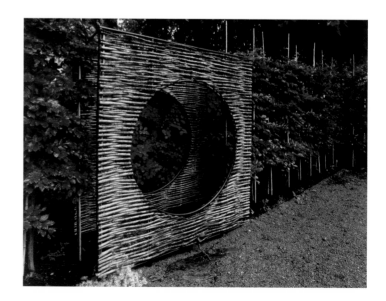

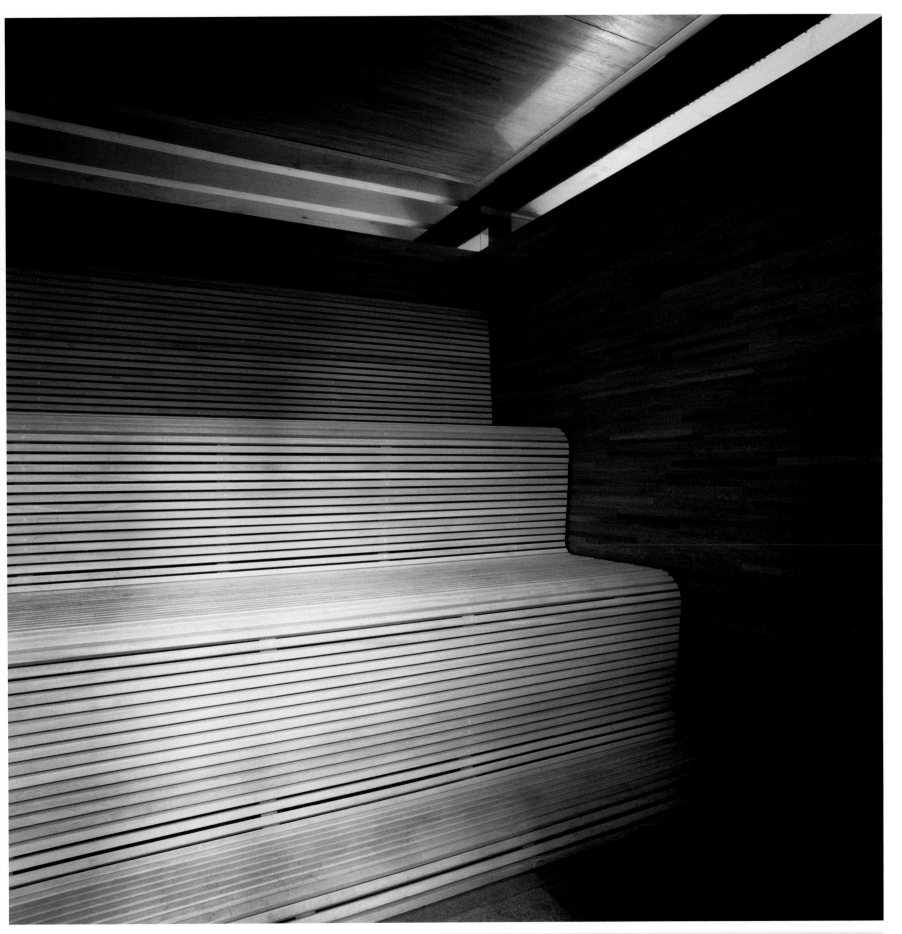

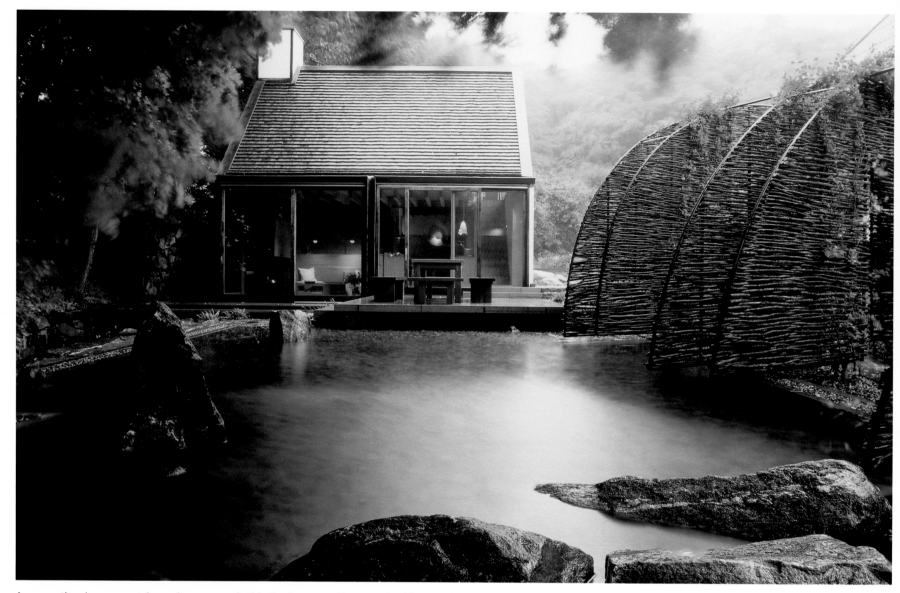

An evocative, Japanese-style garden surrounds this tiny house and bestows it with a magical air.

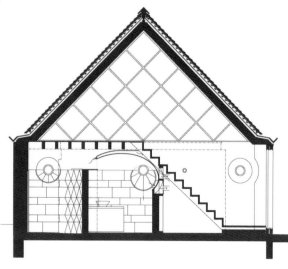

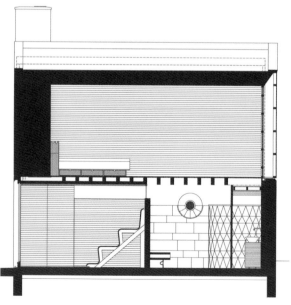

Sections

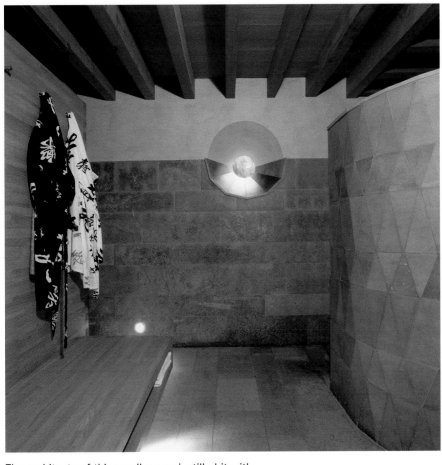

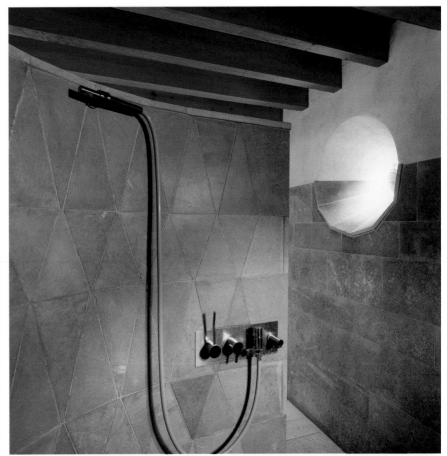

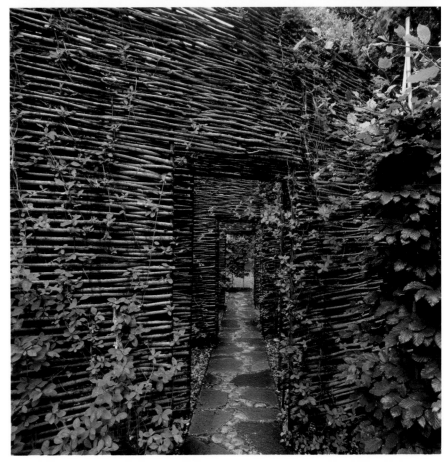

The architects of this small space instilled it with an intimate and quiet ambience through the use of soft lines and warm materials.

A Residence in Küsnacht

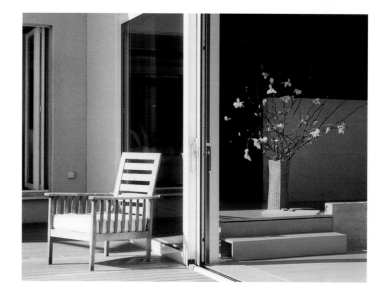

This house, located in a small Swiss village, is characterized by sober shapes and the special way in which it articulates voids. The aim of this project was to eliminate—rather than to add to—architecture. In keeping with this objective, the result is a house of remarkably right angles and light colors, which is additionally flooded with the light that streams in through its large windows. On the top floor of the house, one finds the main bedroom, which has a built-in spa and opens onto a spacious terrace. A low, cement wall serves to separate the bath from the sink. Beyond them, at the other end of the room, the showers are lit from above by a skylight. Exposed cement is a common denominator throughout this Oriental-inspired house.

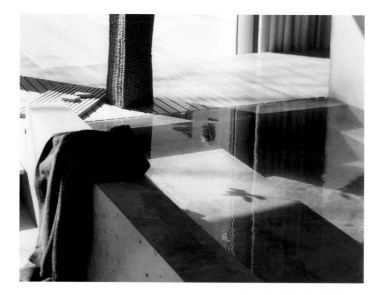

Architect: **Samuel Lerch**
Location: **Küsnacht, Switzerland**
Photos © **Bruno Helbling/Zapaimages**

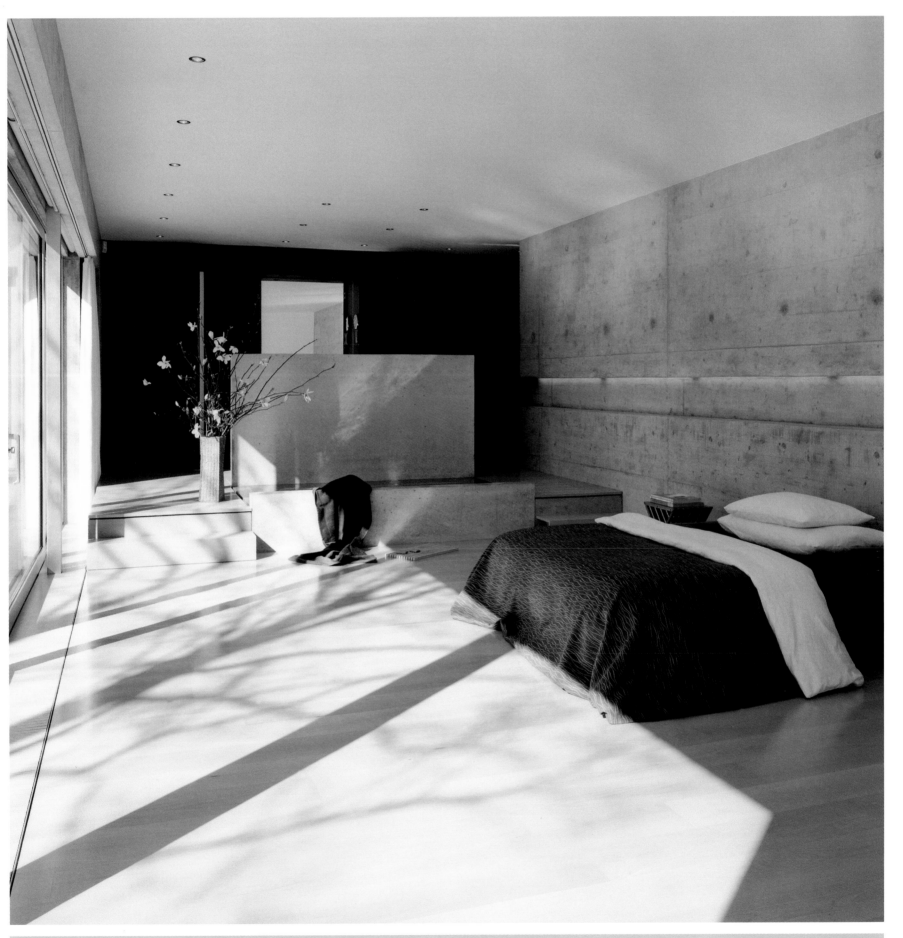

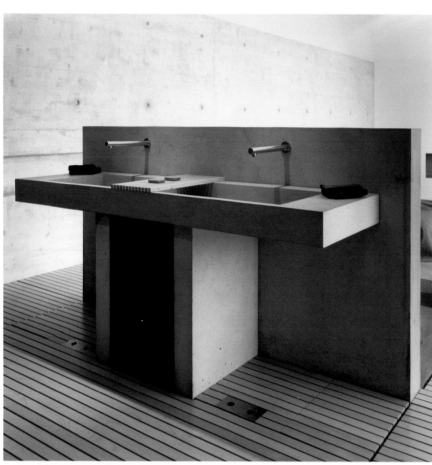

The bath, located next to the bed, is evidence of the owners' interest in enjoying a healthy lifestyle.

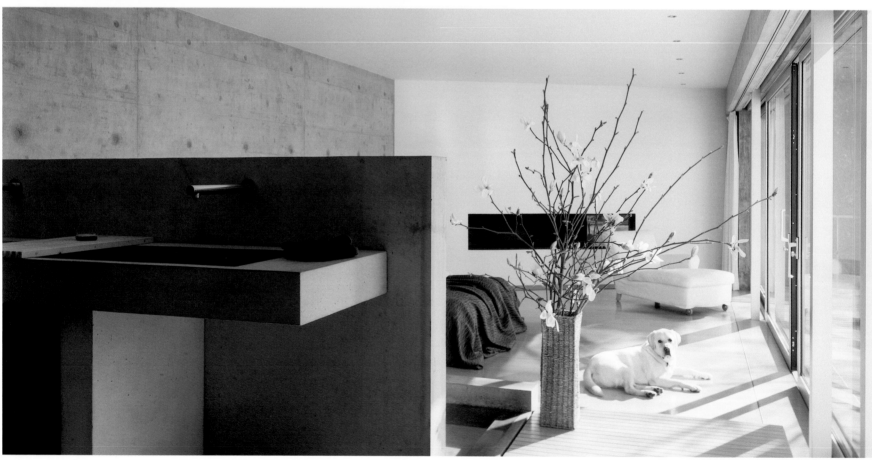

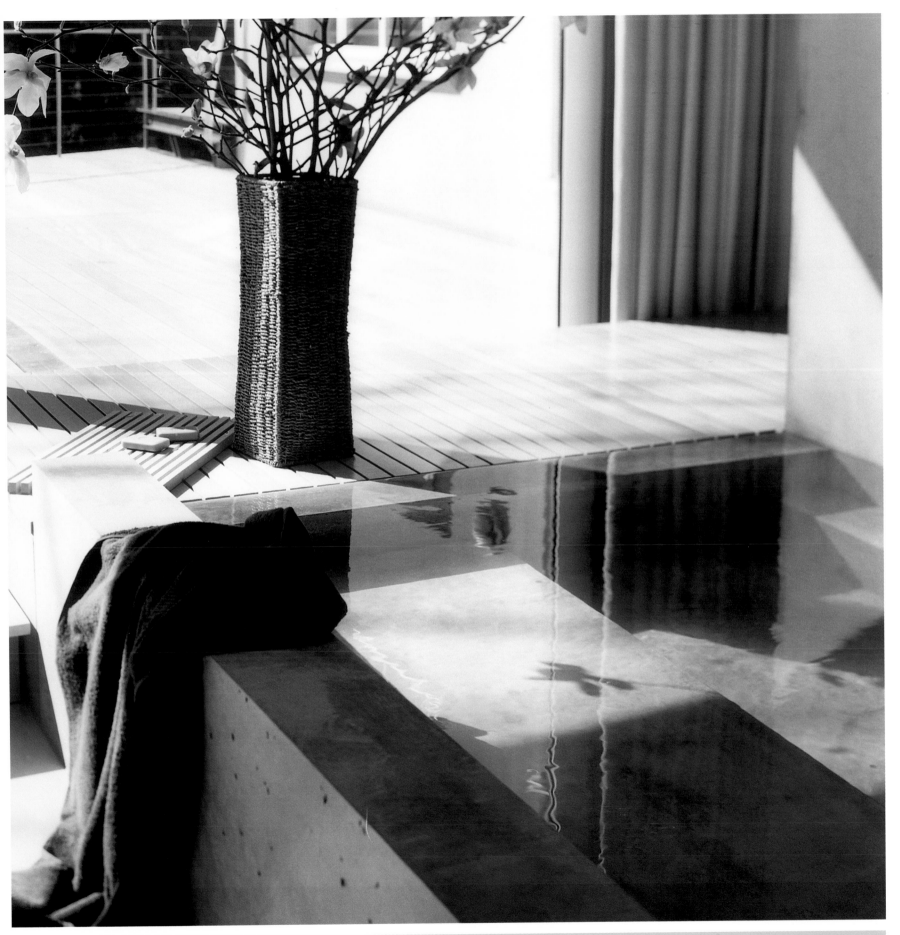

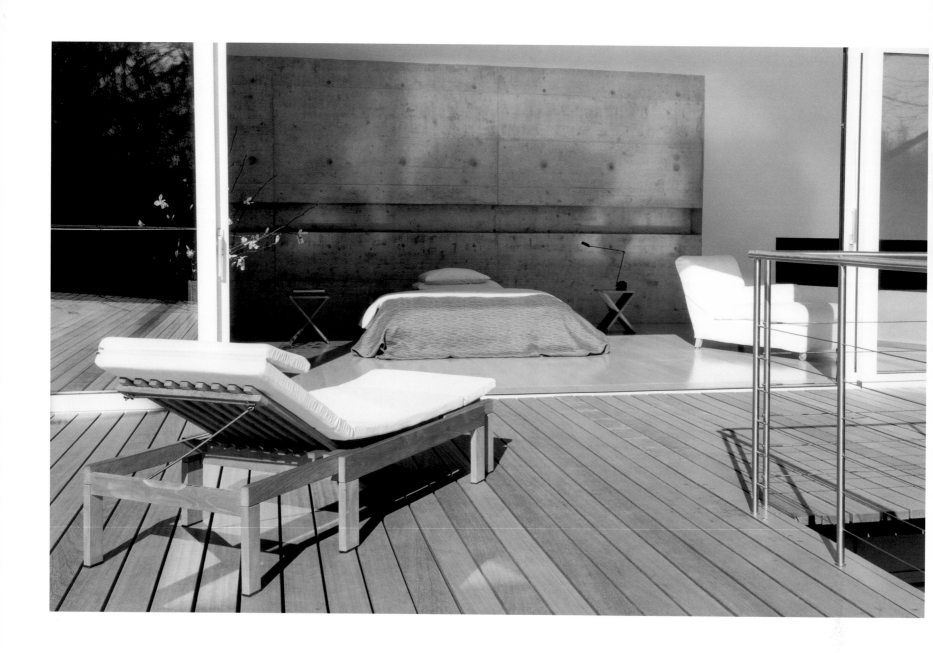

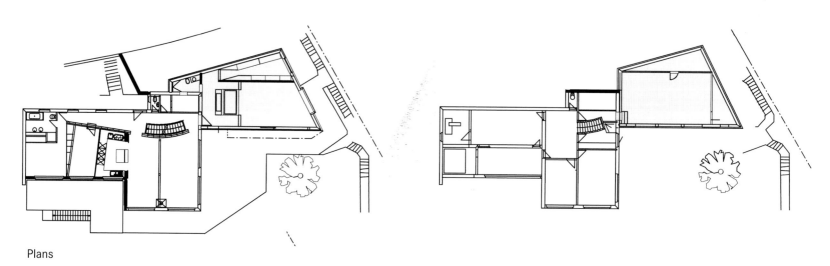

Plans

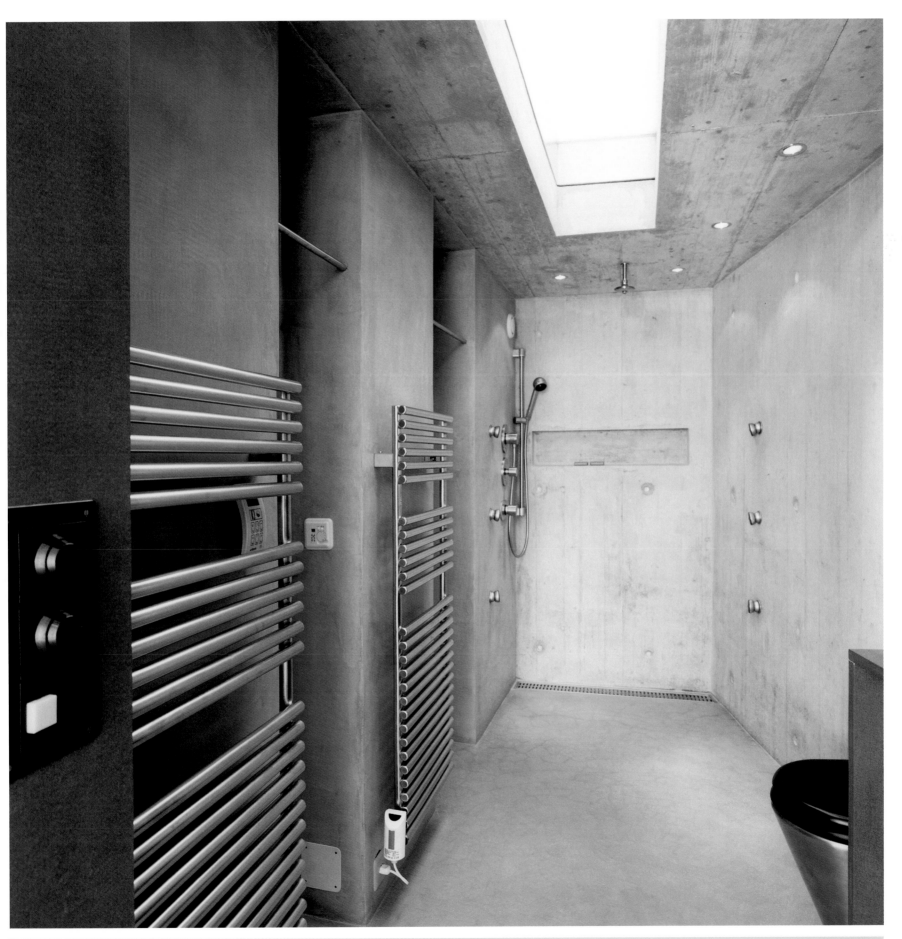

Las Encinas

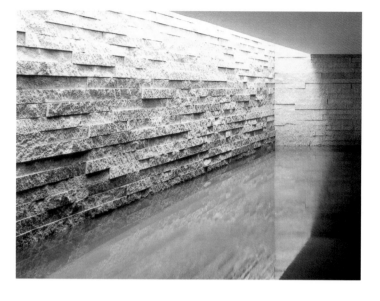

This house, located in a residential area outside Madrid, was conceived of as a giant geode. It is a solid building, sheathed in granite, with two floors aboveground and a basement. No detail was overlooked in its design and construction, and it even has an elevator to connect the various floors. An inner courtyard brings light into different parts of the house, from the vestibule to the covered pool, which is where the spa is located. The walls surrounding the pool are also clad in granite, in contrast to the wooden deck, which was designed to contrast with the cold stone and to make the area more inviting to the touch. A faint light enters through an opening in the ceiling to instill the space with calm, and turns the act of bathing into a unique moment for relaxation and enjoying oneself. There is also a sauna and hydromassage bath, both of which enjoy views out onto the garden.

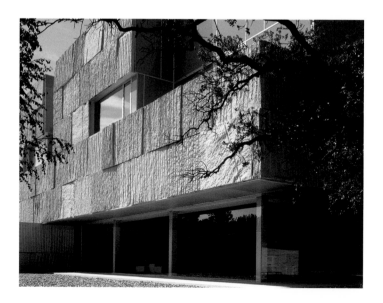

Architect: **Ignacio Vicens and José Antonio Ramos**
Location: **Madrid, Spain**
Photos © **Eugeni Pons**

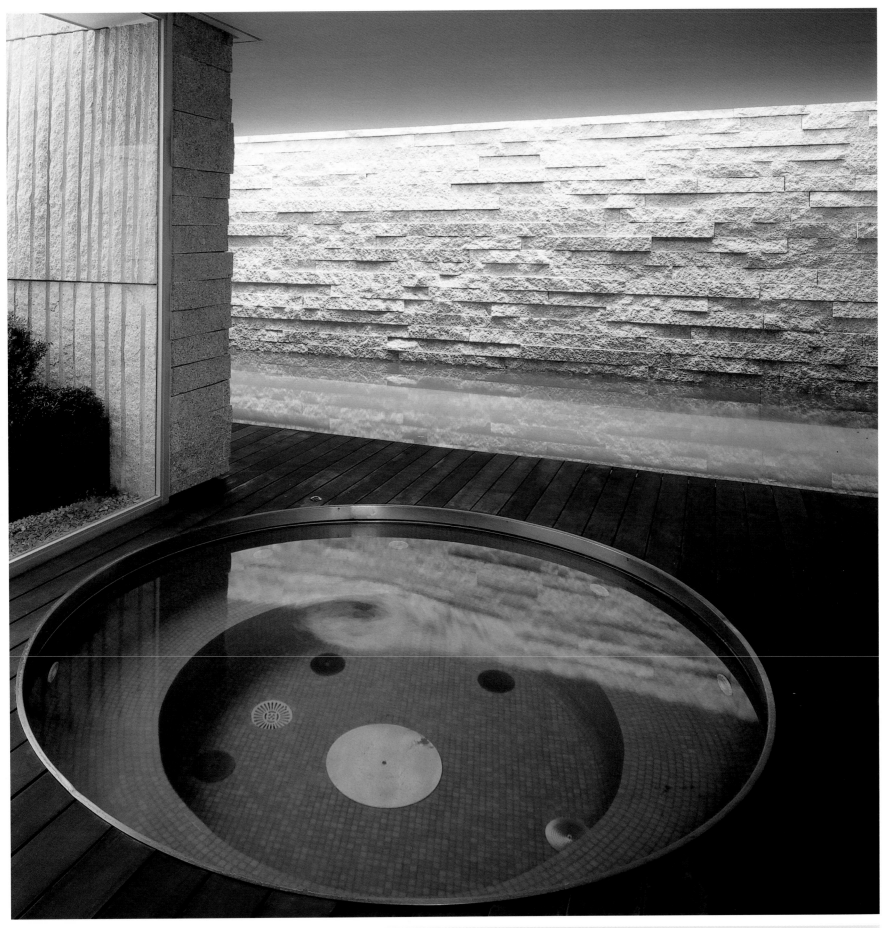

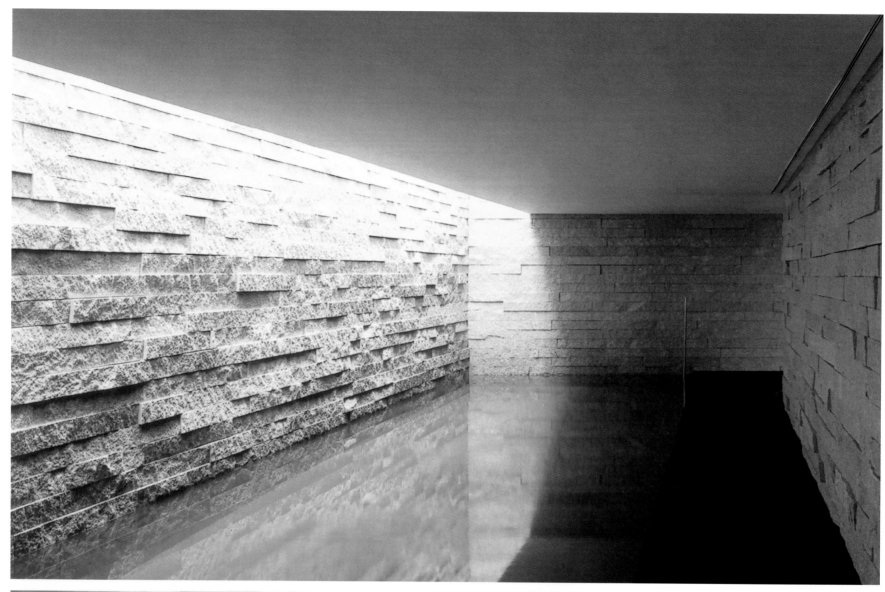

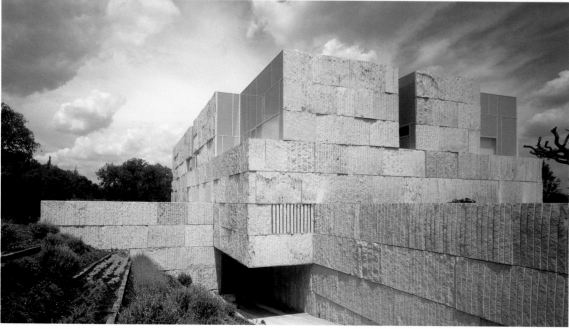

The forcefulness of the stone around the indoor pool contrasts with the softly lit atmosphere and the warmth of the wood details.

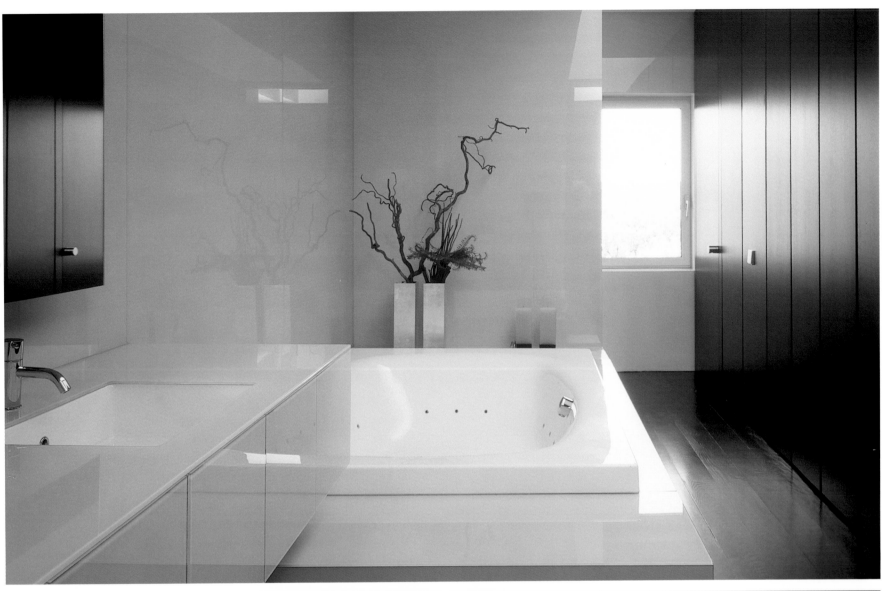

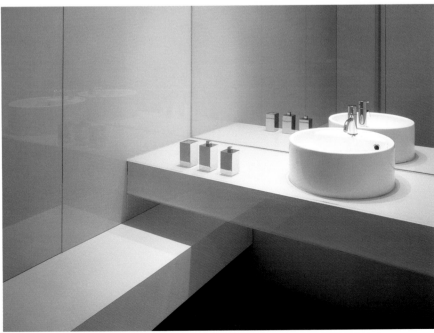

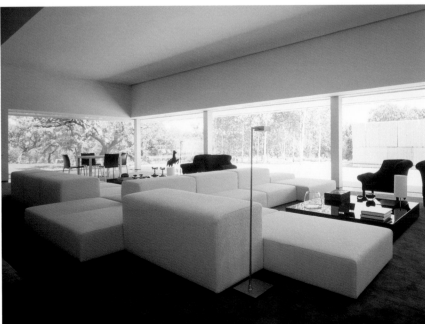

Villa Öjersjö

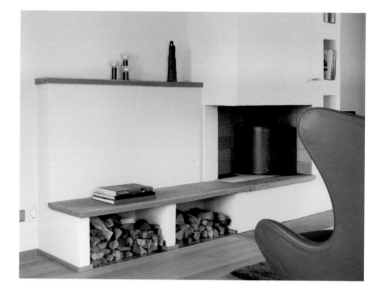

The objective behind the design of Villa Öjersjö was to create a house that would be contemporary, yet warm. Simple lines, and the use of natural light and materials such as glass, wood, and stone, were key to achieving this. The house includes a series of rooms designed to be enjoyed in a social setting, such as the wine cellar/bar in the basement. Other rooms were designed for relaxation and rest, such as the bathroom, with its hydromassage bath and sauna. The bathroom is spacious and modern, and displays a fresh and light-filled aesthetic. The large hydromassage bath distinguishes the space and the tempered glass and white tiles give it a touch of sophistication. The sauna, located in the basement, is a warm and highly intimate space. The contrast is evident: the color black and natural beech define a calmer and more personal space for rest. Saunas are widespread throughout Sweden, and in this home, one can engage in this healthy habit in the best of conditions and with the latest in technology.

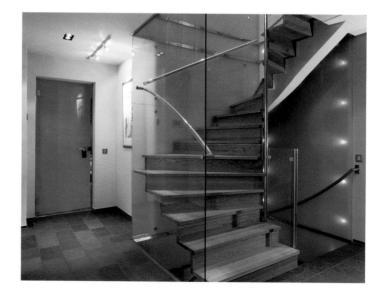

Architect: **Ulf Norr/MFA Kupé Corporation**
Location: **Gothenburg, Sweden**
Photos © **James Silverman**

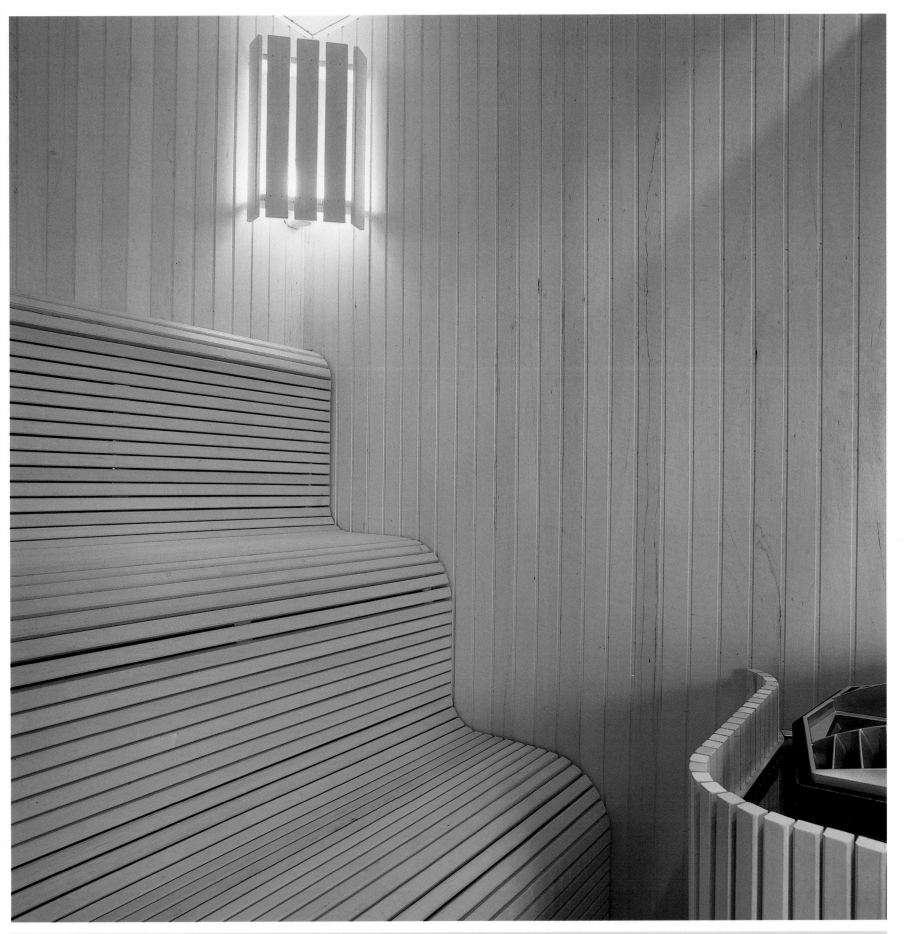

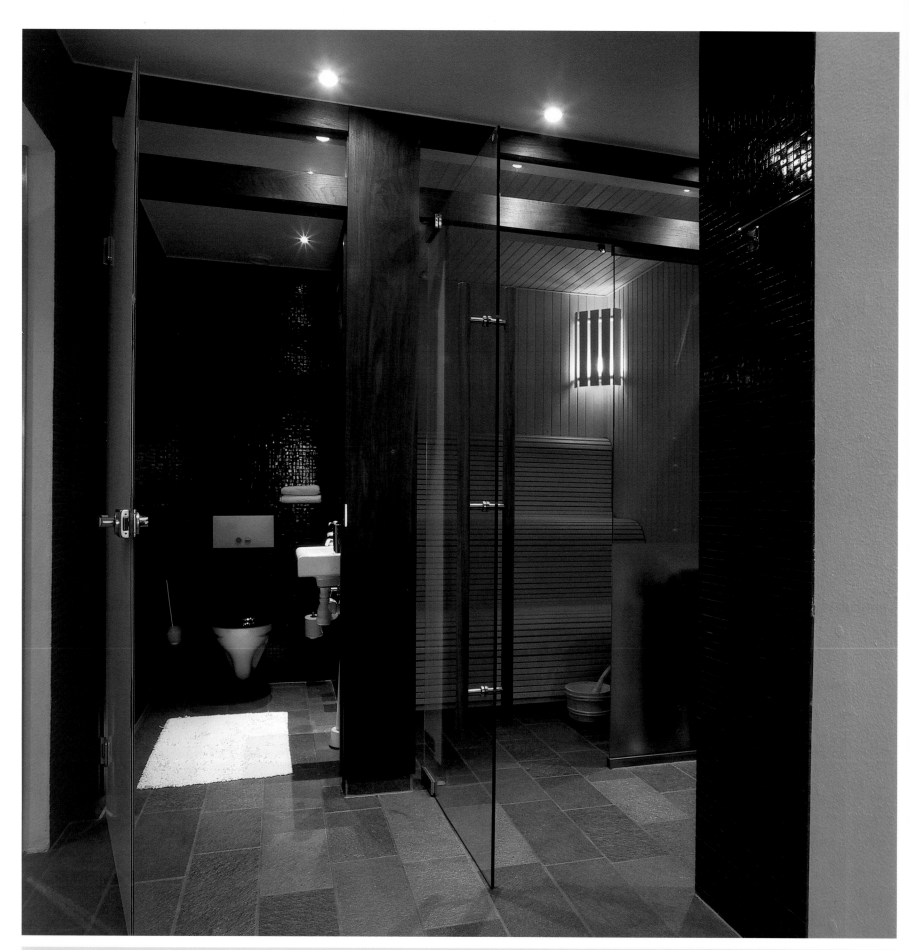

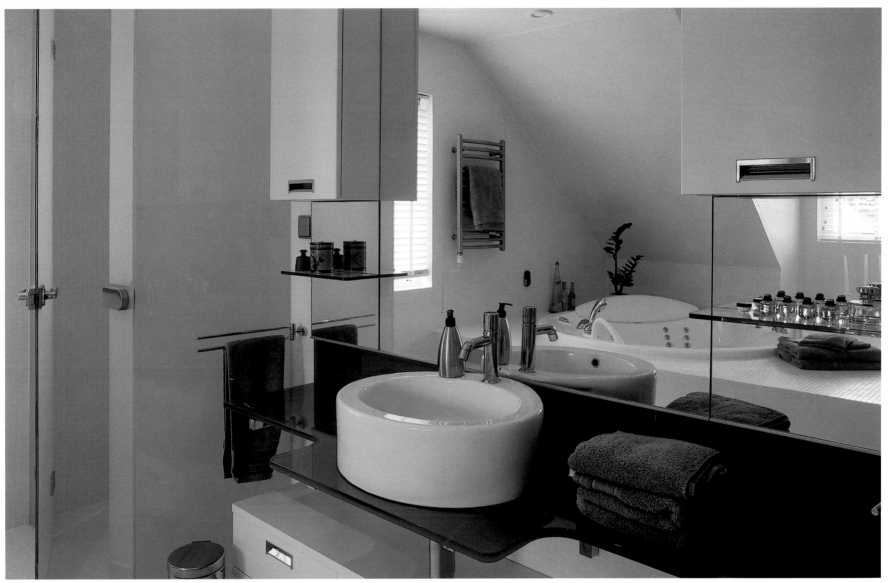

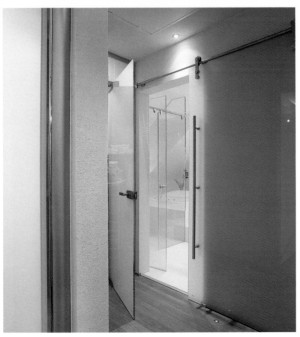

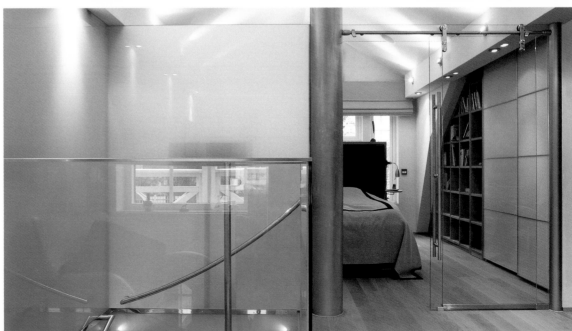

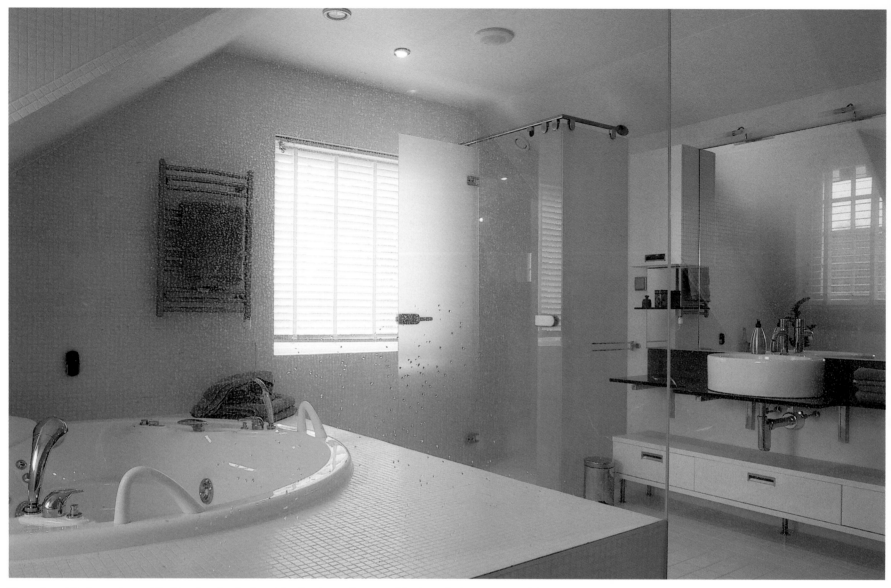

The color white is an element that lends a fresh air and luminosity to the room. The large hydromassage tub is the most important element in the bathroom.

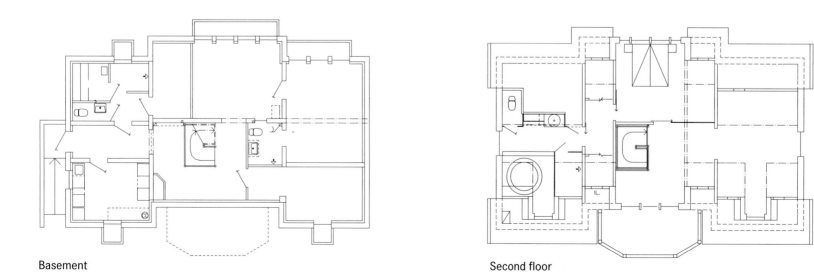

Basement

Second floor

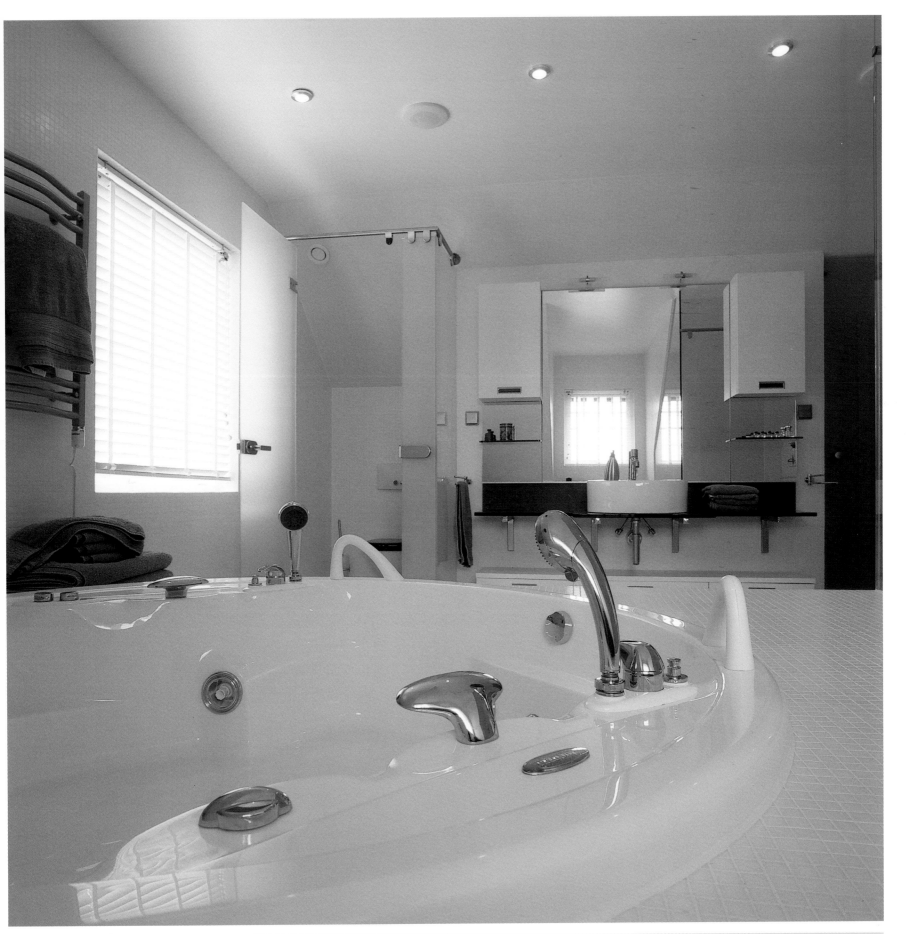

A Duplex in Battery Park

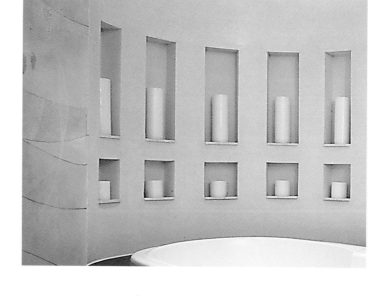

This 2,200-square-foot duplex, located in the financial district of Manhattan, belongs to a young entrepreneur who works in the entertainment industry and had purchased two apartments he aimed to combine into a single residence. His requirements were manifold: in addition to equipping all the rooms with a television and sound system, requiring spacious guest bedrooms and a practical kitchen, he felt it essential that the largest spaces be dedicated to relaxation. In the main bathroom, the bathtub and shower—both of which enjoy a hydromassage—are installed atop a platform. The stage that houses the bathtub has two rows of niches—these were designed to hold candles, which are perfect for imbuing the room with a peaceful air. If the guest should so desire, he or she can listen to music to round out his or her experience. The décor consists of neutral, but warm colors and a thoroughly unique mural.

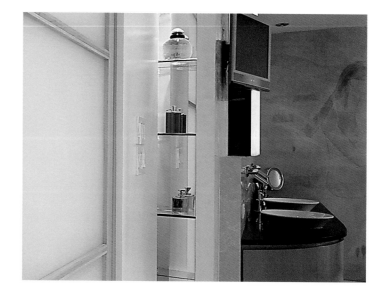

Architect: **Leopoldo Rosati**
Location: **New York City, United States**
Photos © **Leopoldo Rosati**

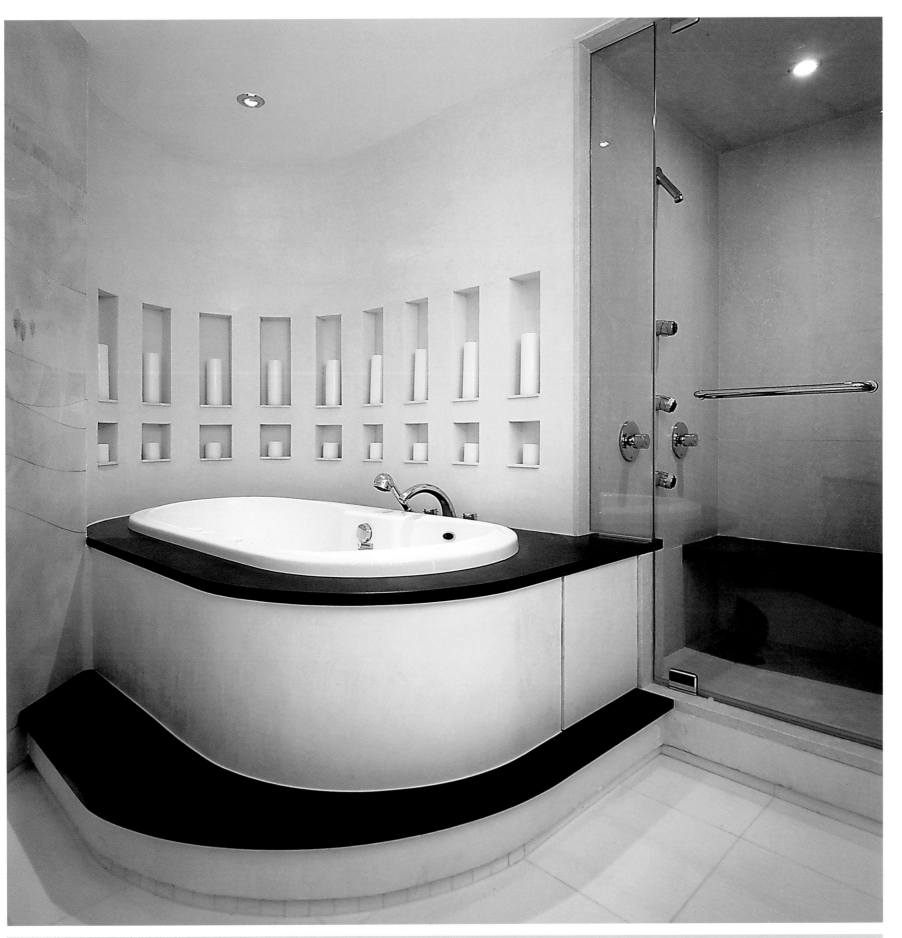

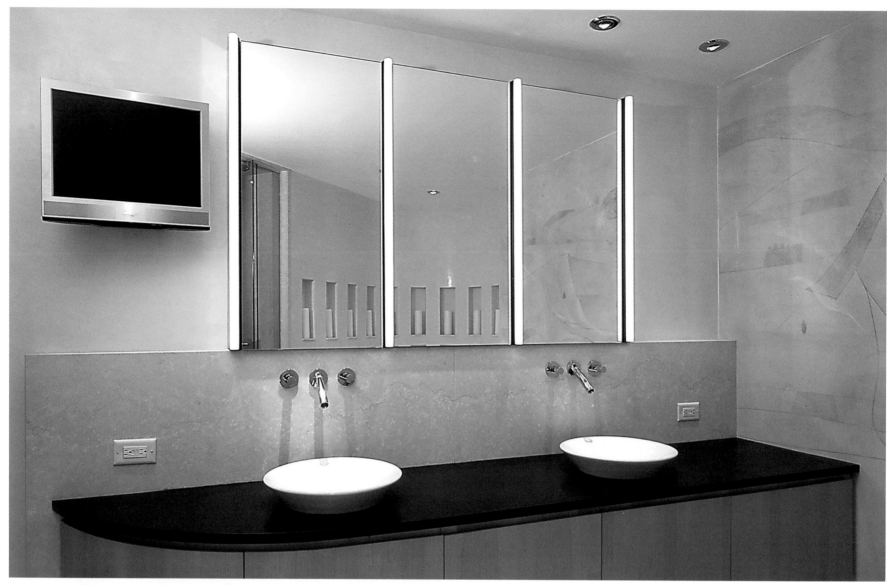

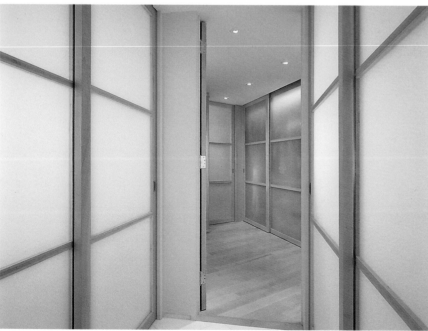

This bathroom has two doors: one from the dressing room that connects to the master bedroom, and a second opening—formed by sliding panels—that opens to the hall.

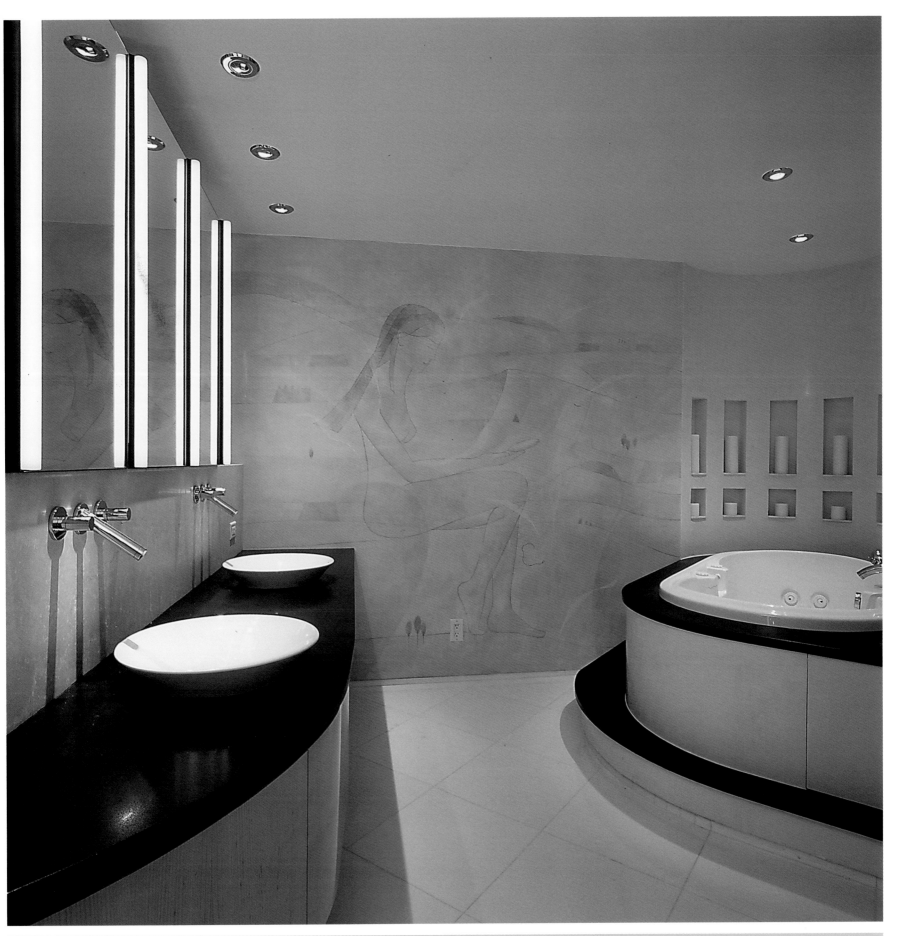

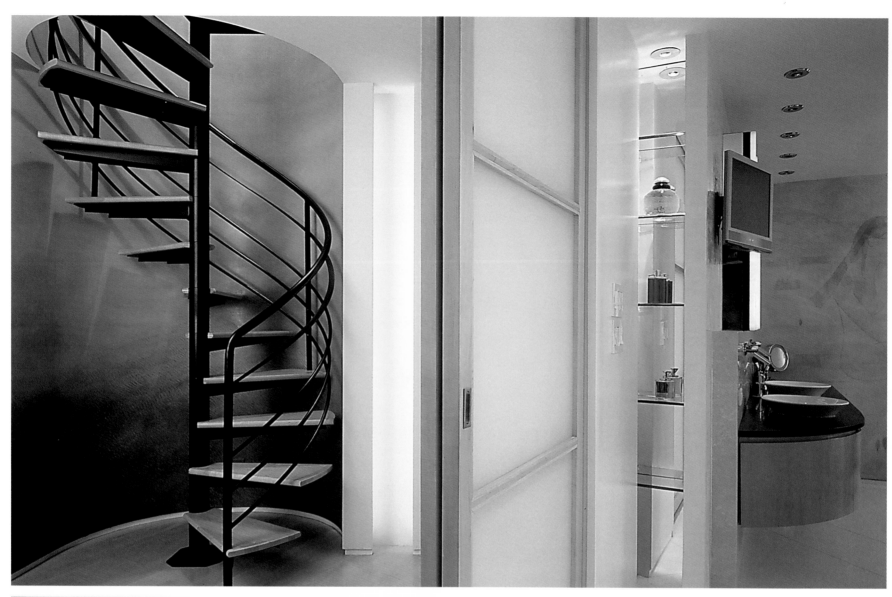

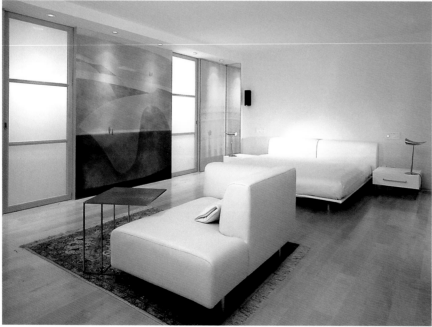

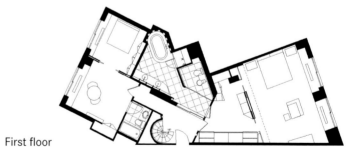
First floor

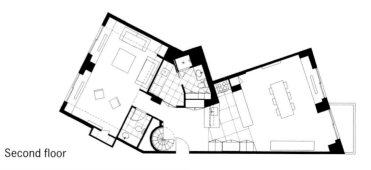
Second floor

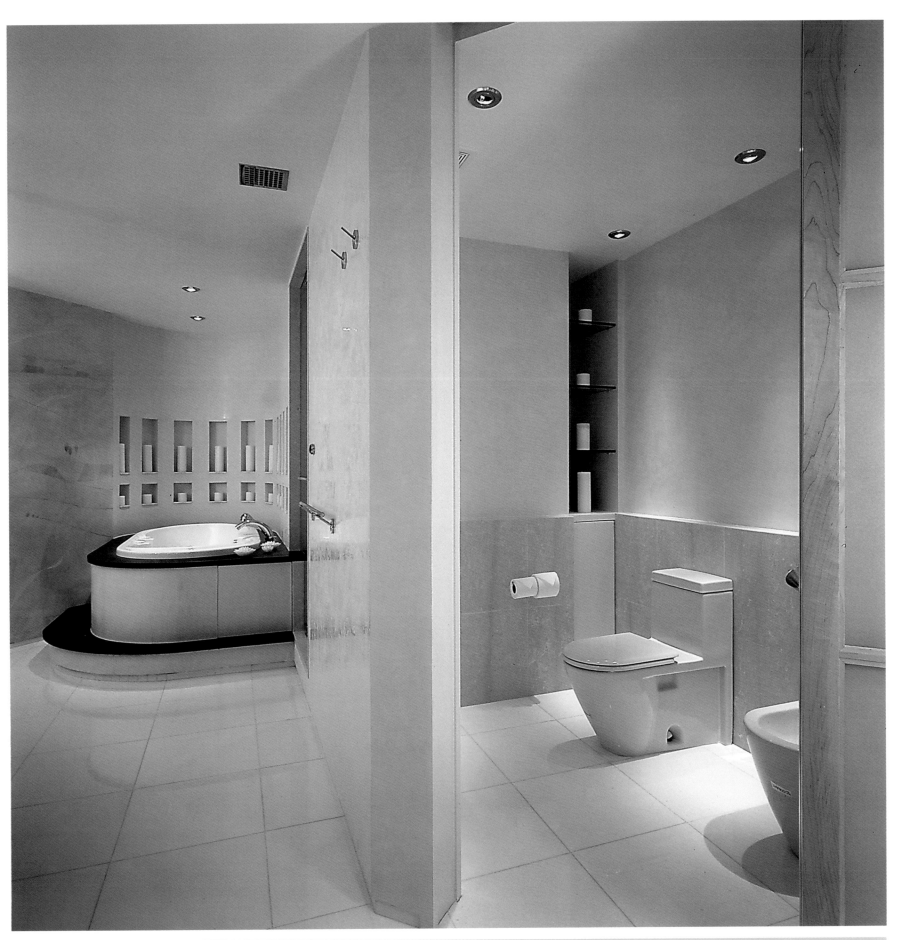

At the End of the Day

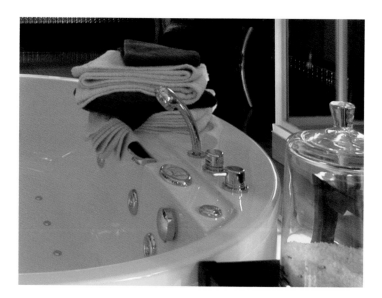

The full range of amenities offered by this spa are arranged into three areas: first, there is a central nucleus dominated by a free-standing hydromassage bath, which appears to float atop of sea of lights; meanwhile, on opposite sides of the bathroom, one finds two showers and two hydromassage cabins; and last, on the remaining two sides, the designers placed the sinks and the toilets. The lighting—in warm or cold light, based on the area—and a meticulous décor spell out a luxurious and extremely comfortable space. The showers are finished in different, "his 'n' hers" materials: the showers are tiled in white tessera for her and in silver for him. The hydromassage cabins, which include options for aromatherapy and chromotherapy, are also freestanding. The lighting system on the ceiling, which is programmable, further enhances the ambience of the room—which is fitted entirely with equipment furnished by Ideal Standard—and provides a perfect place to achieve physical and mental equilibrium.

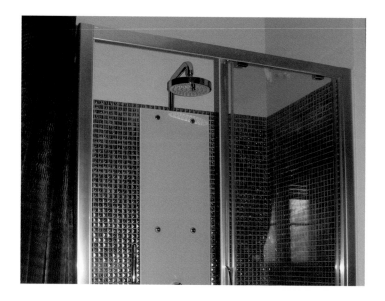

Decorator: **Raquel Chamorro for Ideal Standard**
Location: **Madrid, Spain**
Photos © **Fernando Coma/Ideal Standard**

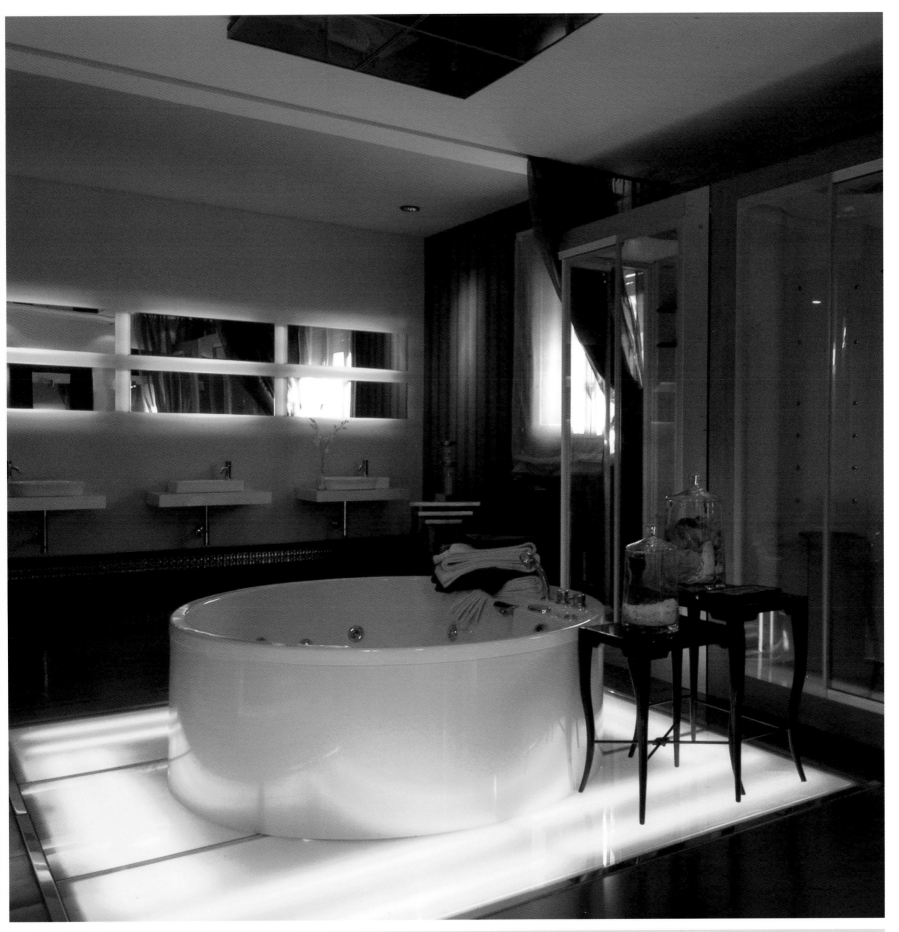

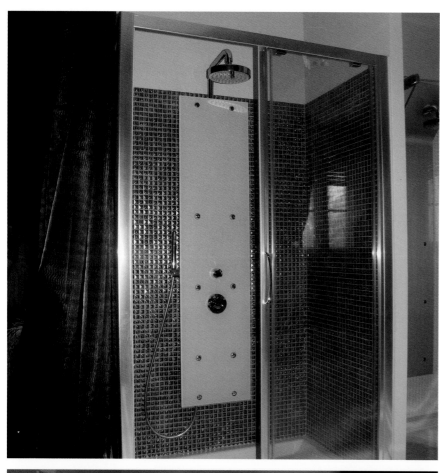

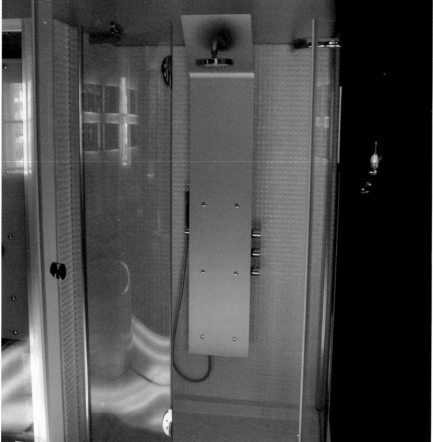

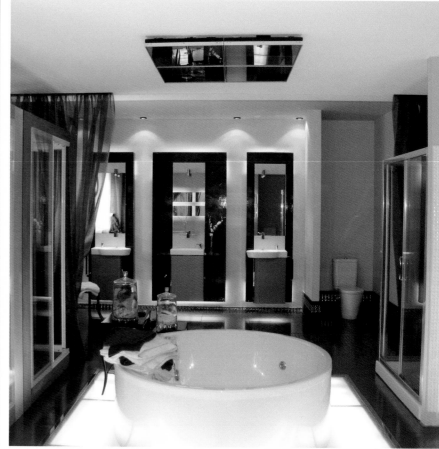

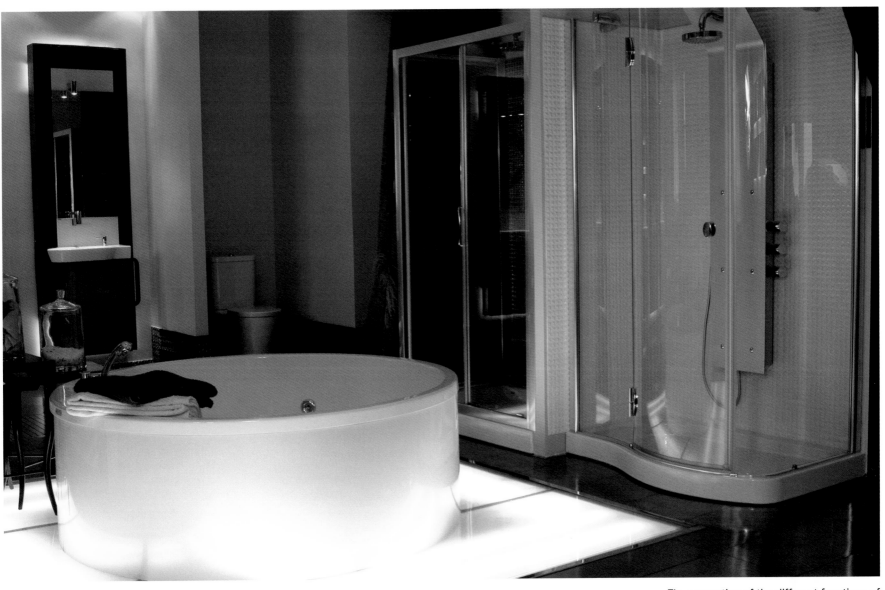

The separation of the different functions of the spa allows one to enjoy a wide variety of treatments based on one's preferences; anything from hydromassage to a steam bath, or even chromotherapy, is available.

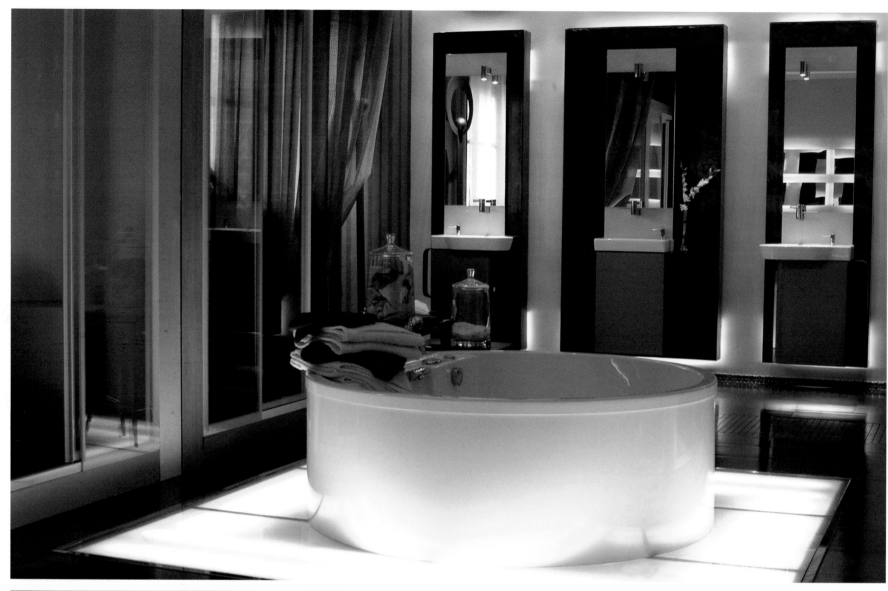

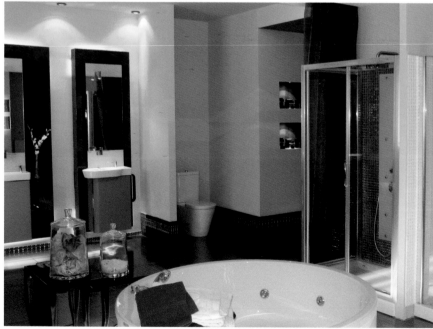

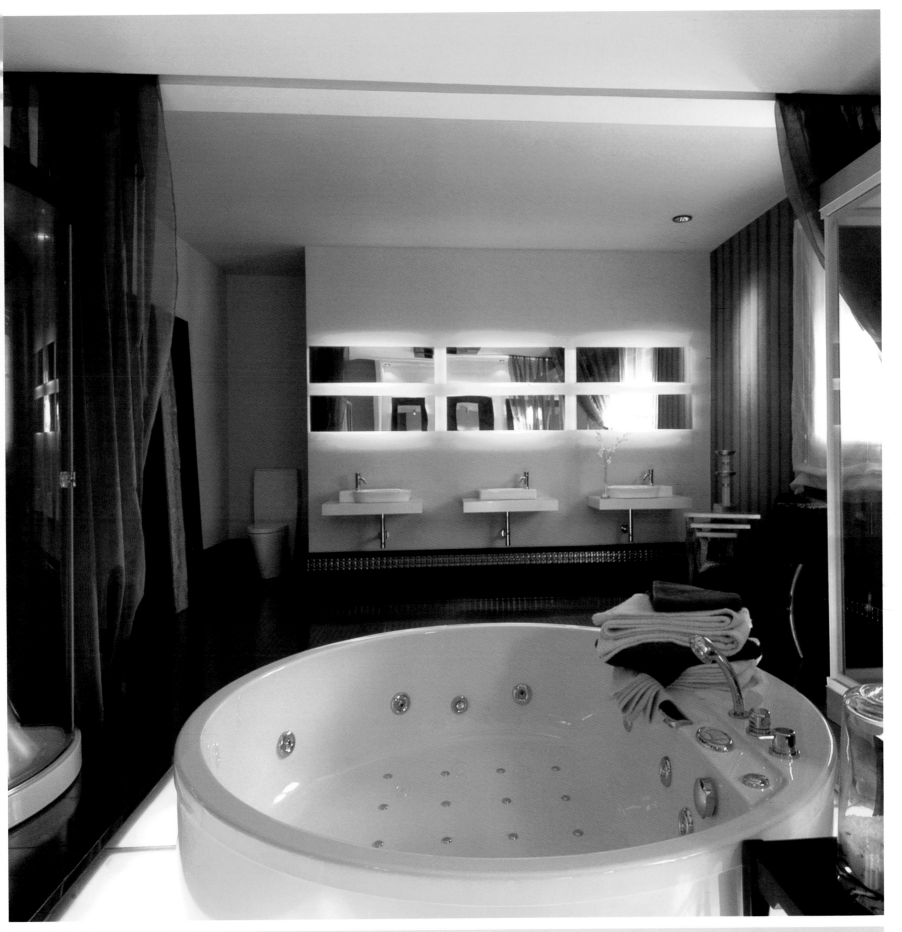

T Residence

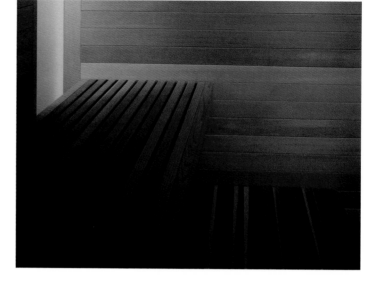

The renovation of this bathroom aimed to create a private atmosphere in which space would be unified by the textures of the walls and floor. Designed to represent water flowing from one end of the bathroom to the other, the tiles are different shades of blue and gray and comprise the element that unifies a series of spaces separated by glass panels. Some of these panels were designed to be translucent, for reasons of privacy. Horizontally placed cedar planks were used on the walls and ceiling, which makes the interior seem larger than it is. In one corner, a frosted glass panel allows natural light to enter the house without detracting from the privacy of this space, in which speakers let one listen to music. This, in sum, is a place for relaxing and revitalizing one's body and for dedicating time to oneself.

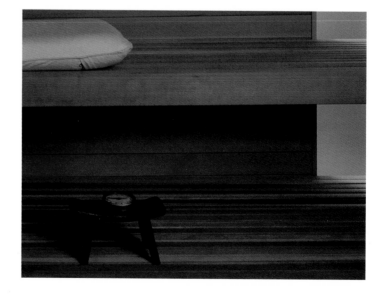

Architect: **Studio Rinaldi**
Location: **New York City, United States**
Photos © **Wade Zimmerman**

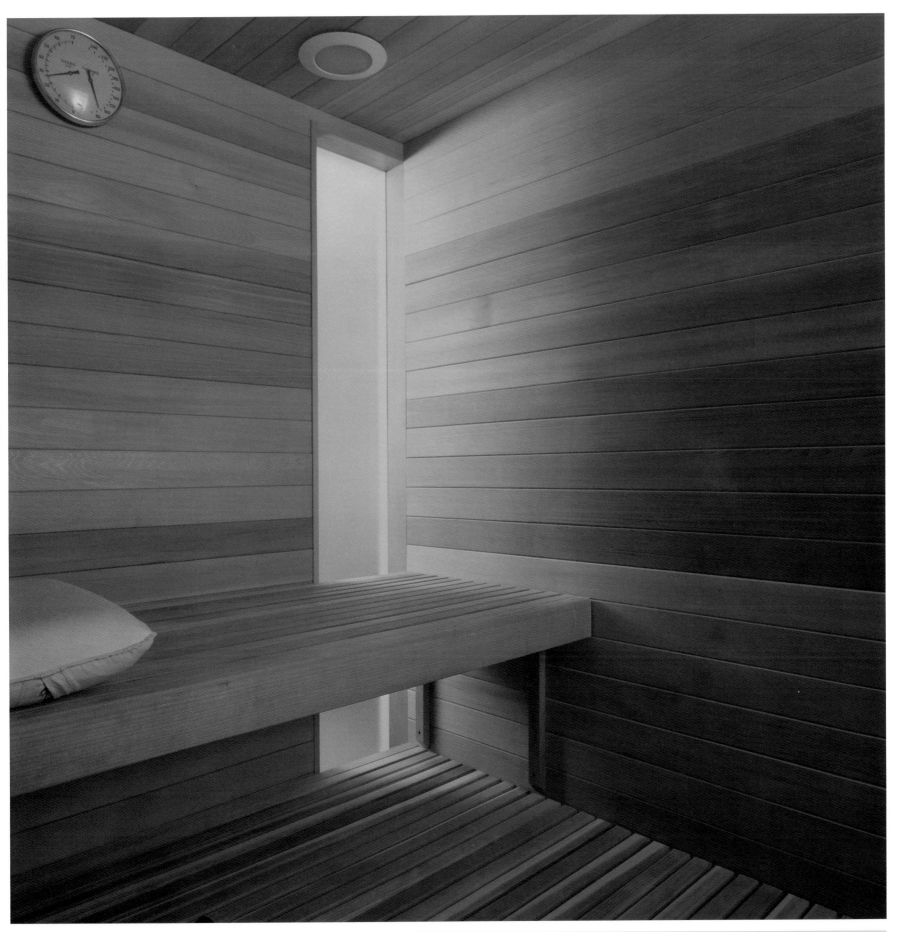

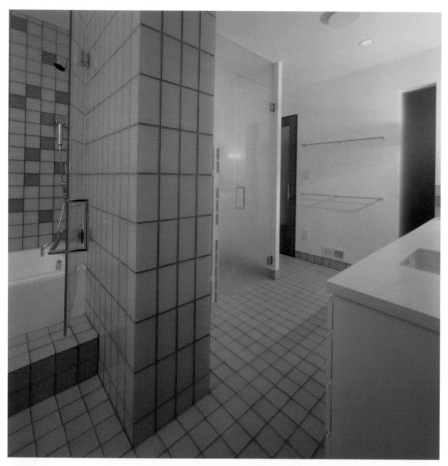

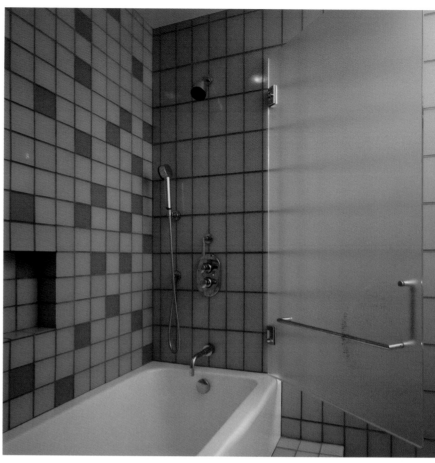

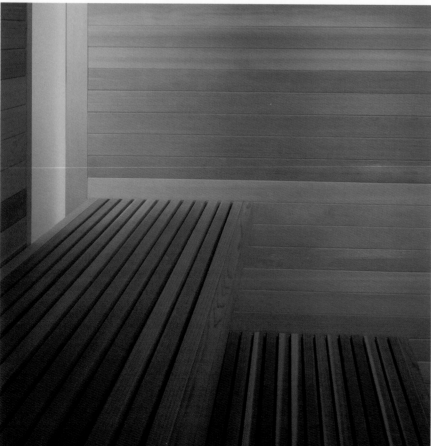

One of the aspects that distinguishes this project is the quality of its finishes and materials, which lends the space a unique elegance.

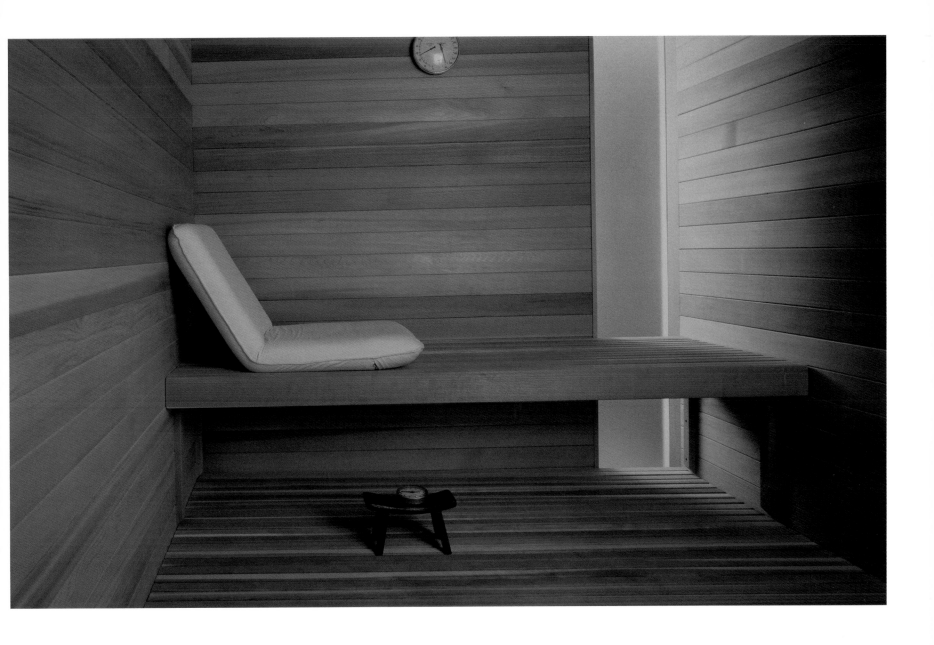

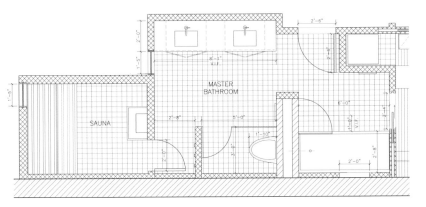

Plan

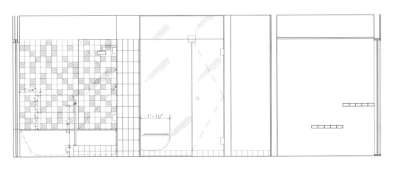

Section

Breuer-Lundberg Getaway

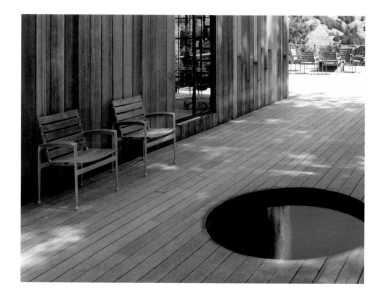

This small getaway, designed by architect Olle Lundberg, is located amid a dense forest of fir trees, which fosters an unrivaled sensation of calm and well-being. It is located two hours outside of San Francisco, and measures just 1,100 square feet, though its spacious terrace makes it seem larger. In its construction, only materials that had been salvaged from other projects were used. The most important two elements are a circular pool 25 feet in diameter and 14 feet deep, and, situated alongside it, a hot-water bath; both of these are fitted into what had served as water tanks for cattle. The simplicity of this house helps it to blend into a landscape in which moon-filled nights transform its pools into black voids and create a magical retreat for the soul. The architect was also in charge of building the house, and has plans to add a sauna that will further enhance the well-being of the owners of this thoroughly natural getaway.

Architect: **Olle Lundberg/Lundberg Design**
Location: **Sonoma, California, United States**
Photos © **J.D. Peterson**

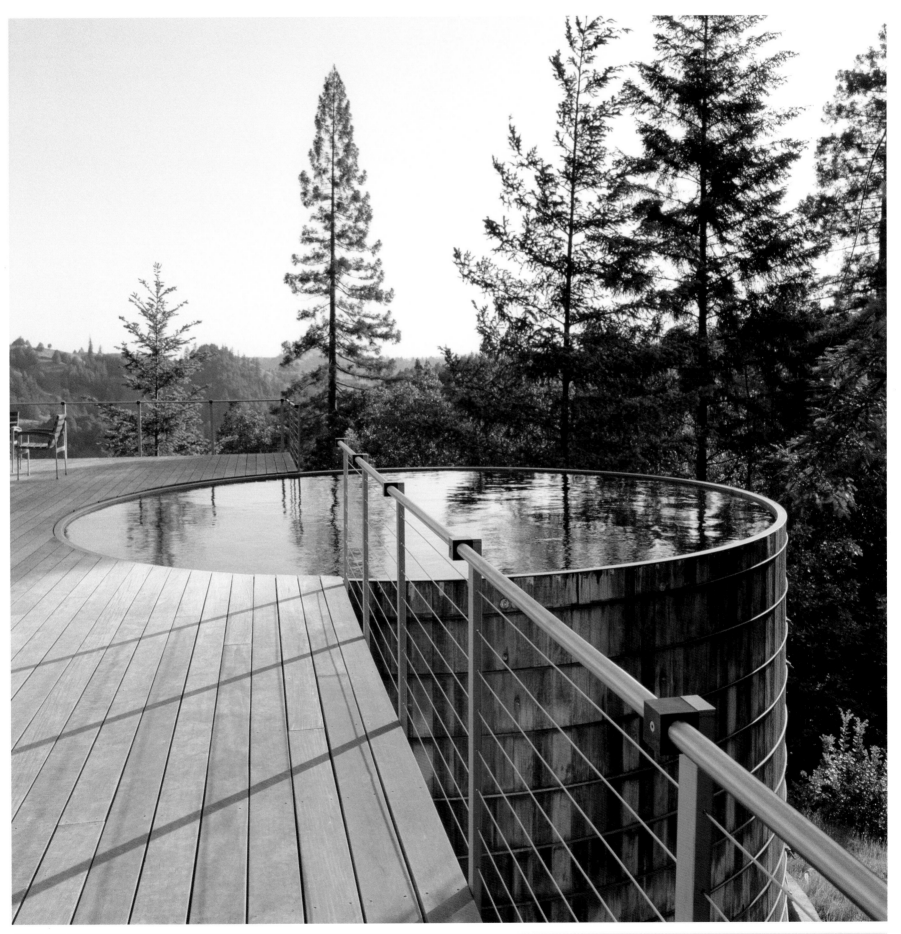

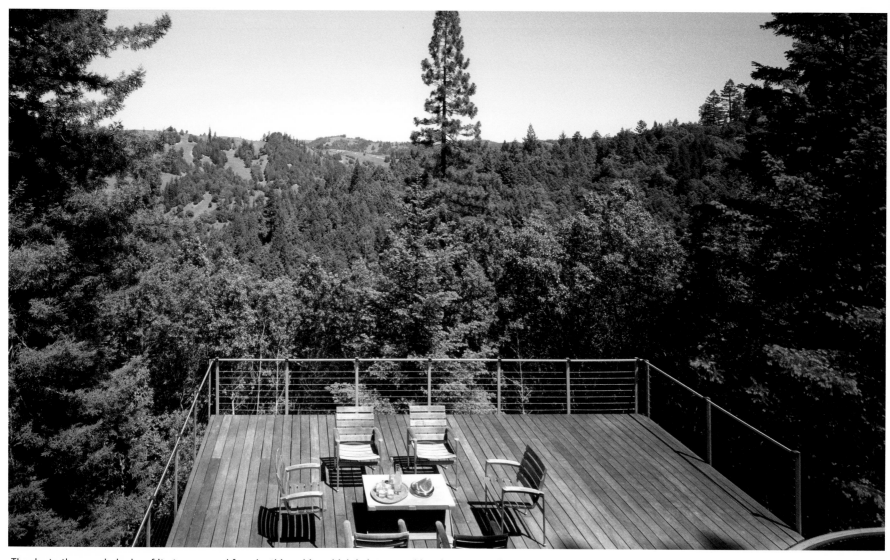

Thanks to the wood planks of its terrace and façade, this cabin, which is integrated into its surroundings, enjoys a warm and comfortable atmosphere.

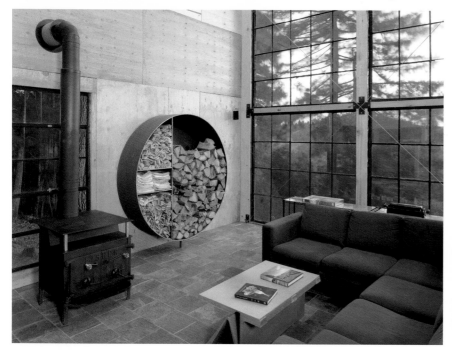

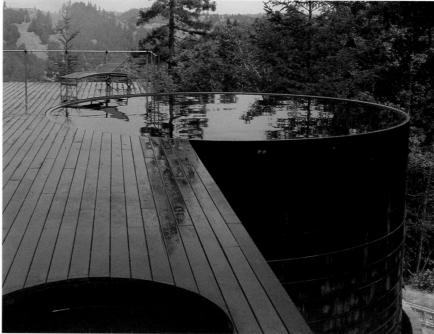

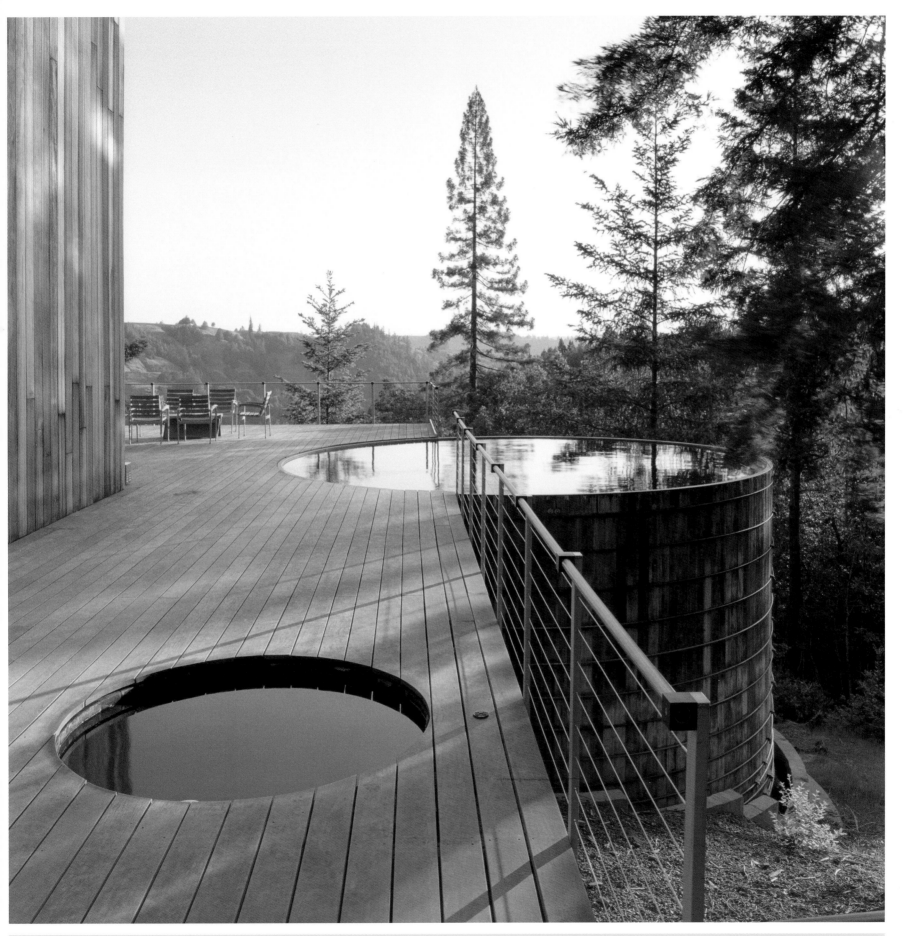

BR House

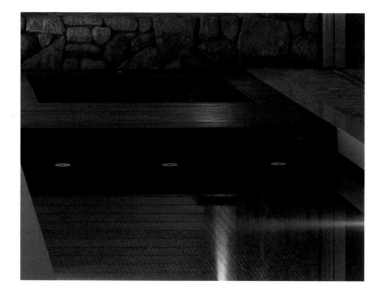

On a breathtaking site in the mountainous region outside Rio de Janeiro, the BR House's spa opens onto the forests that surround it. The upper floor of the dwelling is supported atop a smaller volume—which houses the spa—and two rows of steel columns clad in wood. The main façade of this level is made up of three sliding glass panels that span an opening over 60 feet long. When designing the layout of the spa, the architect respected an enormous rock that rose from the site, and even went so far as to clad the walls in a type of stone quarried locally. Wood abounds in the thermal installations—sauna, hydromassage bath, and pool—alongside neutral and earth tones, which fill the space with warmth. A window in the sauna allows one to make out the hydromassage bath and the entire length of the pool, as the three are aligned in a row. At night, the area is lit by a series of lights located at strategic places on the ground and walls, which creates a diffuse light in the spa and rounds out this sophisticated and elegant atmosphere.

Architect: **Marcio Kogan**
Location: **Araras, Brazil**
Photos © **Nelson Kon**

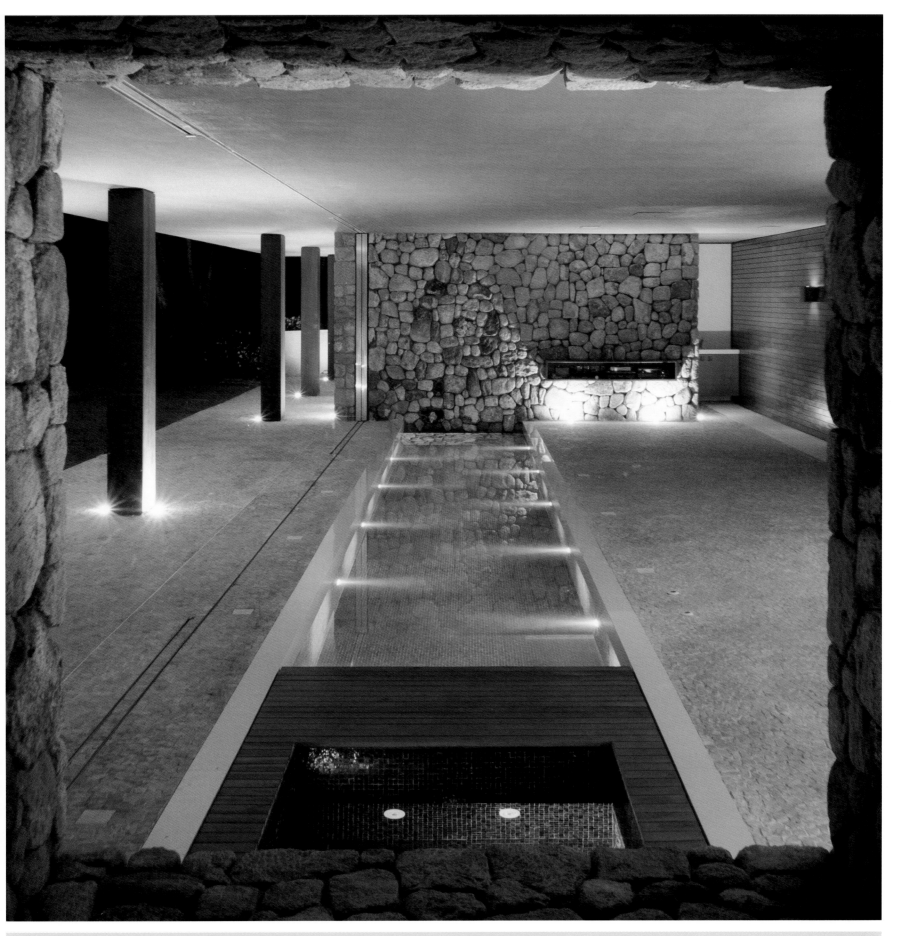

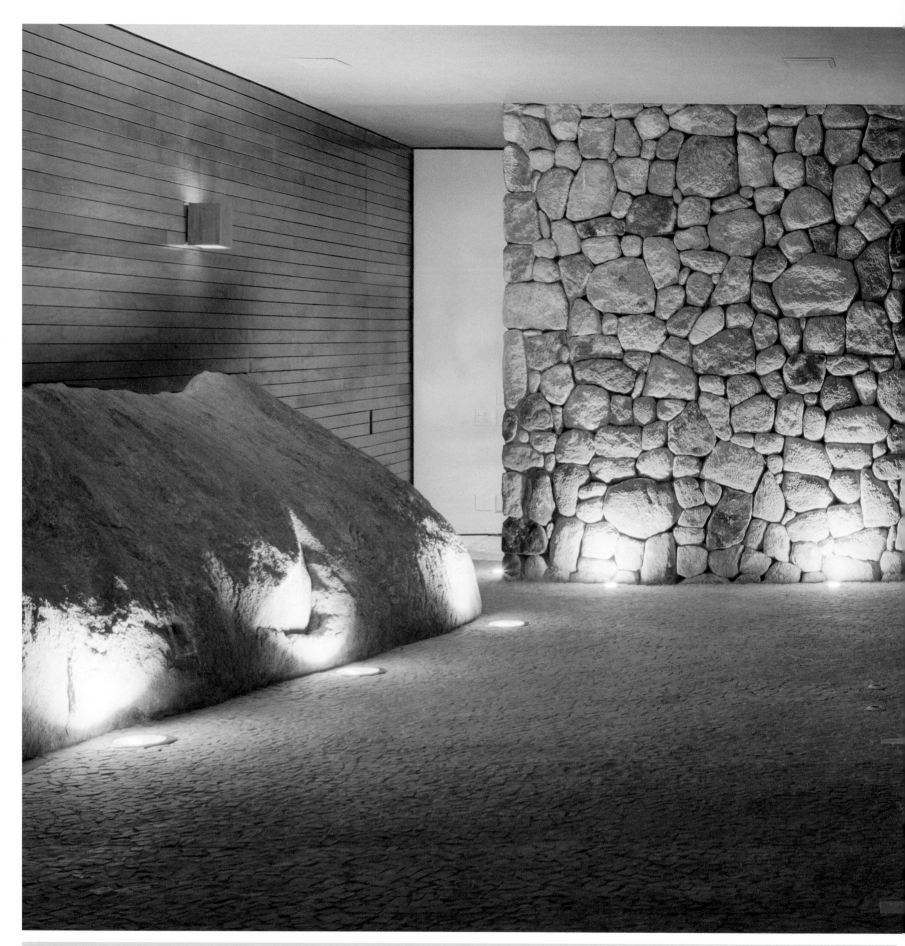

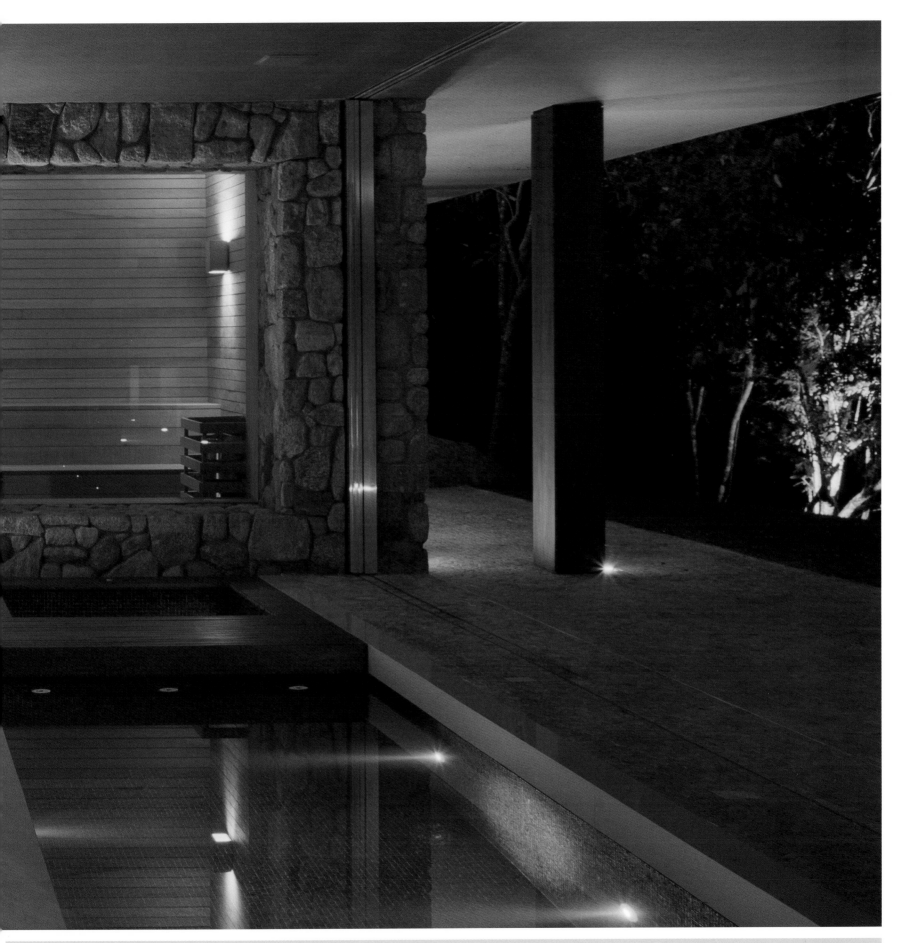

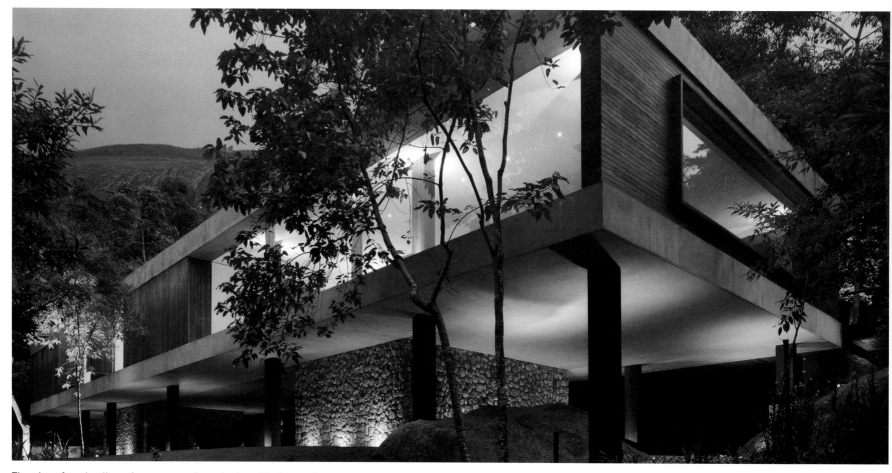

The glass façade allows for a sense of continuity with the outdoor space and causes the sensation of the spa being located under a porch.

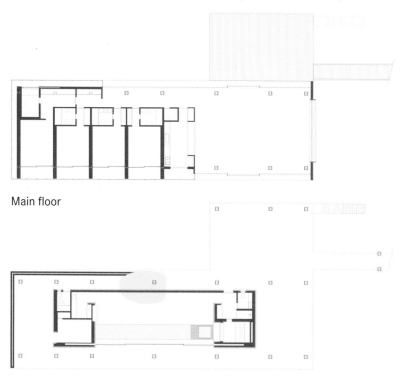

Main floor

Terma floor

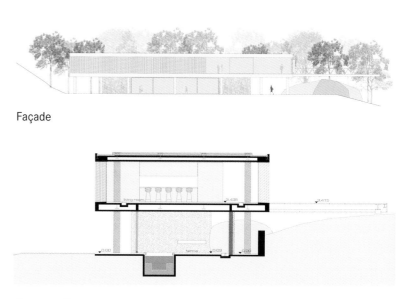

Façade

Cross section

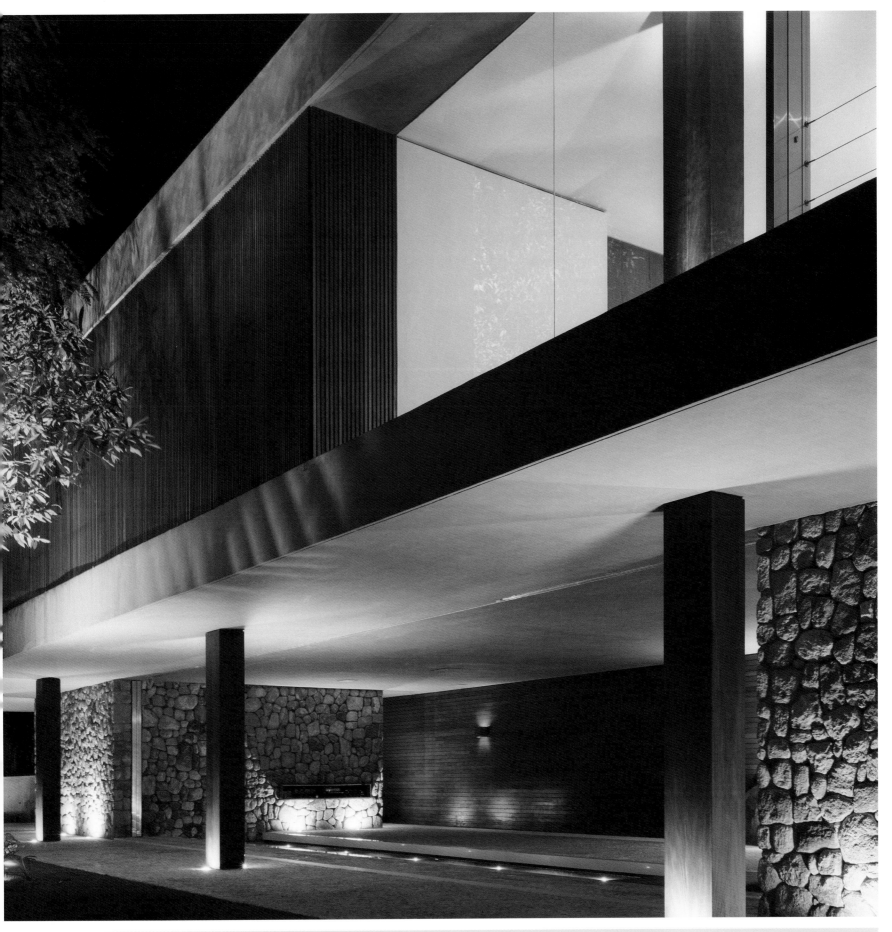

An Apartment in Stockholm

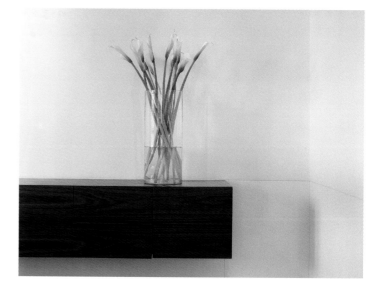

The structure of this almost 3,200-square-foot residence had to be completely redesigned in order to create a work area. This redistribution, then, foresaw gathering all the rooms into the center of the apartment and reserving the sides for circulation. Thus, the bathroom was also placed in the central space, which yields a highly dynamic result featuring two main elements: a sauna and a sizable, white, oval-shaped bath. The exterior structure of the sauna is finished in walnut, which is repeated in other furnishings throughout the house, while the interior is clad in Abachi wood, which is commonly used in these types of installations. On one of the sides, a large window fills the interior with light and allows what would otherwise be a closed space to have access to the bathroom. The bright whites of the décor and the straight lines of the furniture add a dash of minimalist aesthetic to the room.

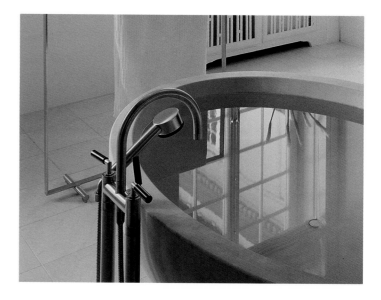

Architect: **Claesson Koivisto Rune Arkitektkontor**
Location: **Stockholm, Sweden**
Photos © **Åke E:son Lindman**

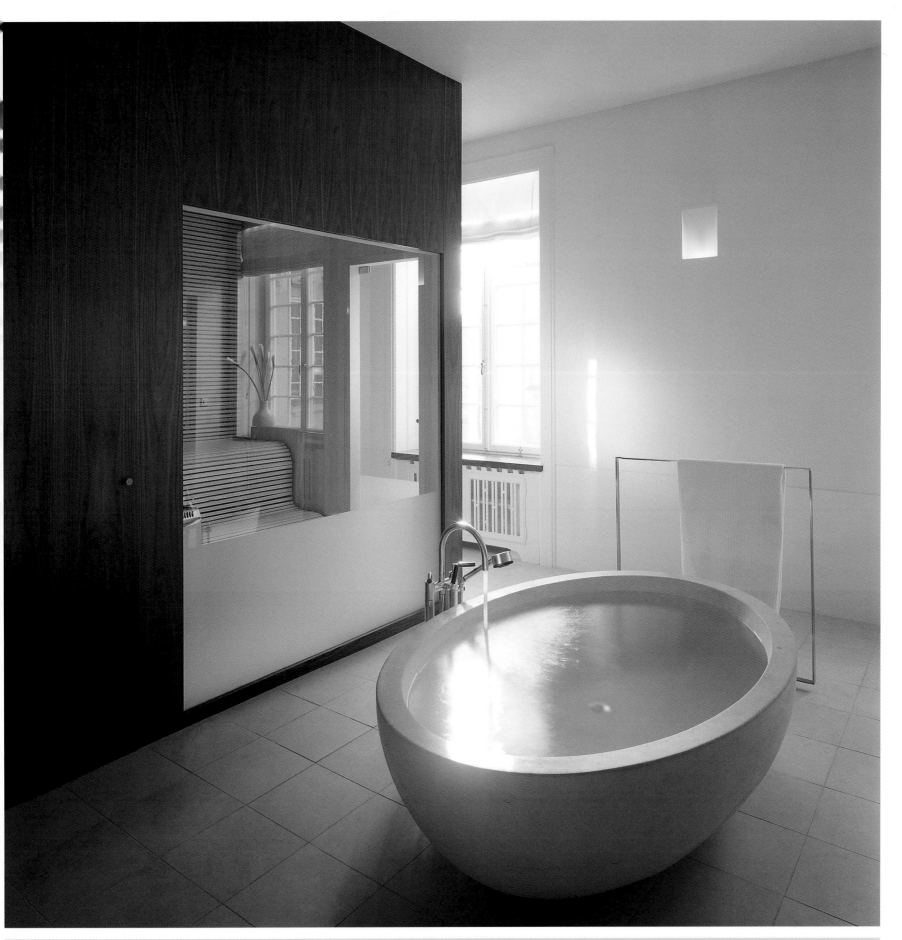

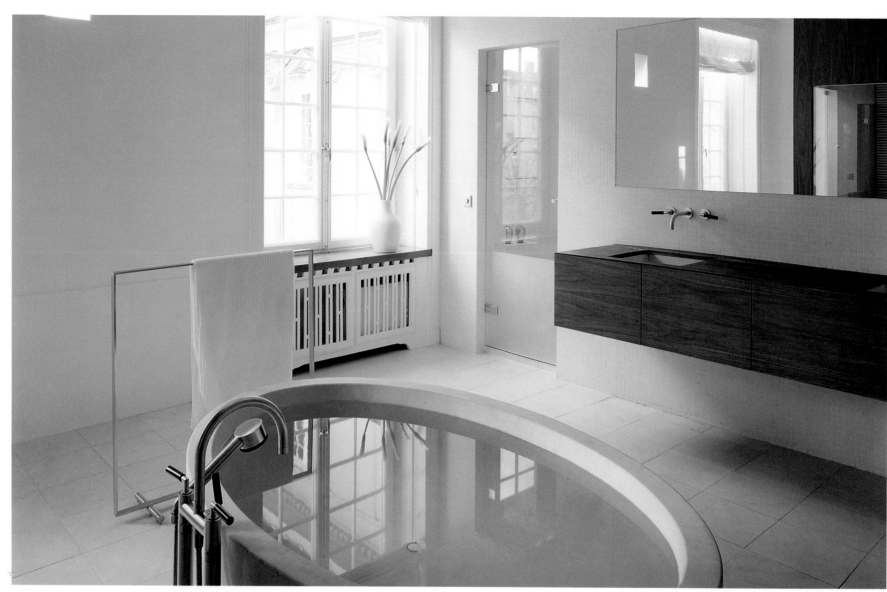

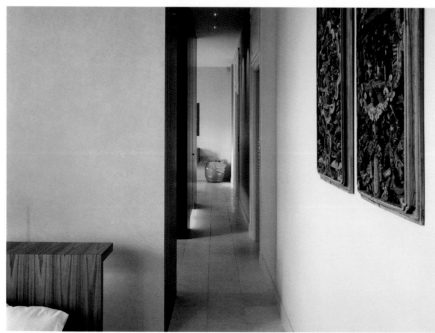

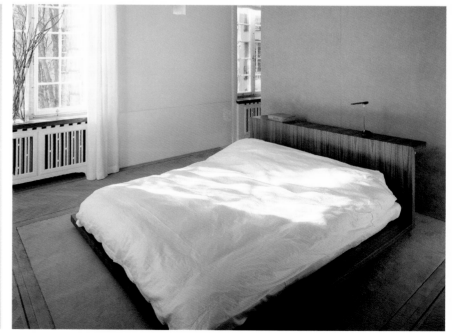

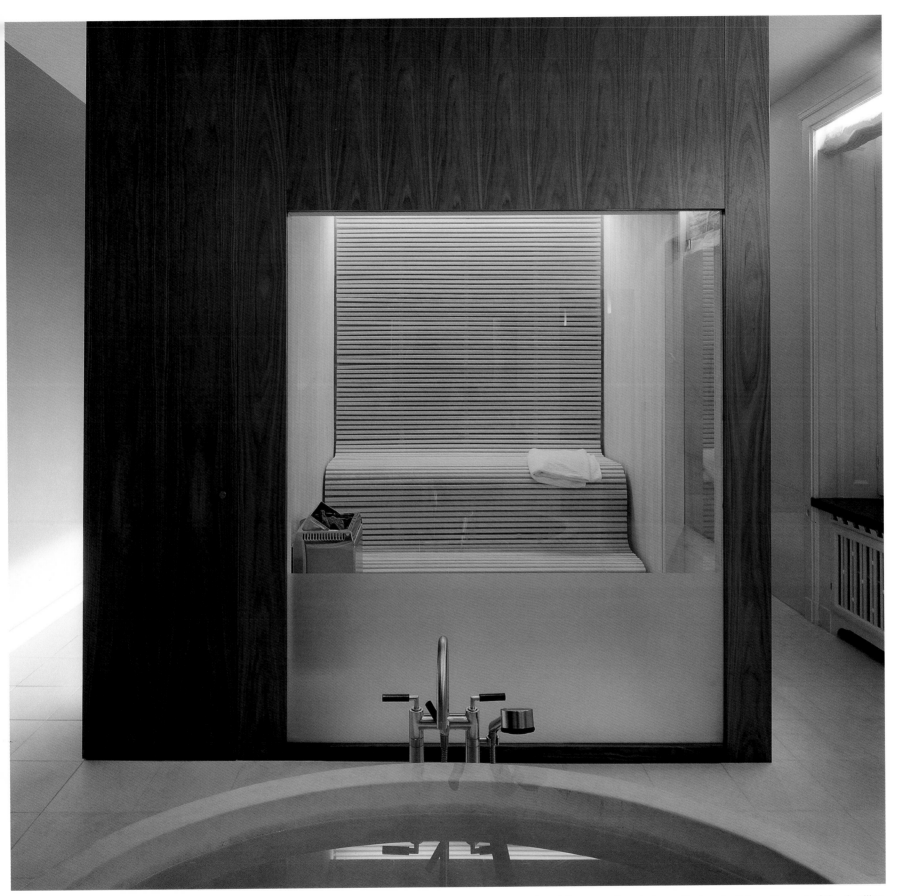

A glass wall in the sauna allows for a certain spatial continuity and keeps the interior of the sauna from being entirely cut off from the rest of the dwelling.

Villa +

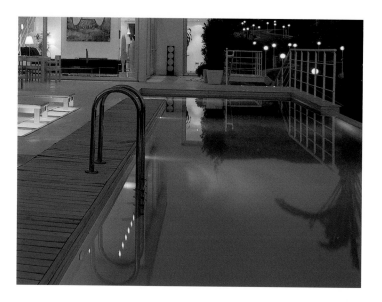

The elements that comprise the bathroom suite in this house are arranged in a row, in which the different facilities are arranged in order of ascending privacy. The shower, which is also designed to serve as a steam bath, is clad in glass tiles and is set back next to the toilet and the bidet. Following in line, one finds the sink, followed by the room that houses the hydromassage bath. The latter is precisely what transforms this bathroom into a unique space, as a spectacular set of windows establishes a visual connection between the bath and a quiet corner of the garden. Thus, while taking a bath, one can enjoy the exterior, which is dominated by spectacular views of the Mediterranean. The entire bathroom is finished in Capri marble, which is similar to the marble used throughout the rest of the house—this establishes a common thread throughout. Elegance and simplicity—along with plenty of light—pervade the house in its entirety.

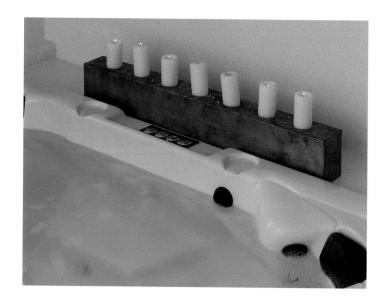

Architect: **Jaime Sanahuja**
Location: **Oropesa del Mar, Castellón, Spain**
Photos © **Joan Roig**

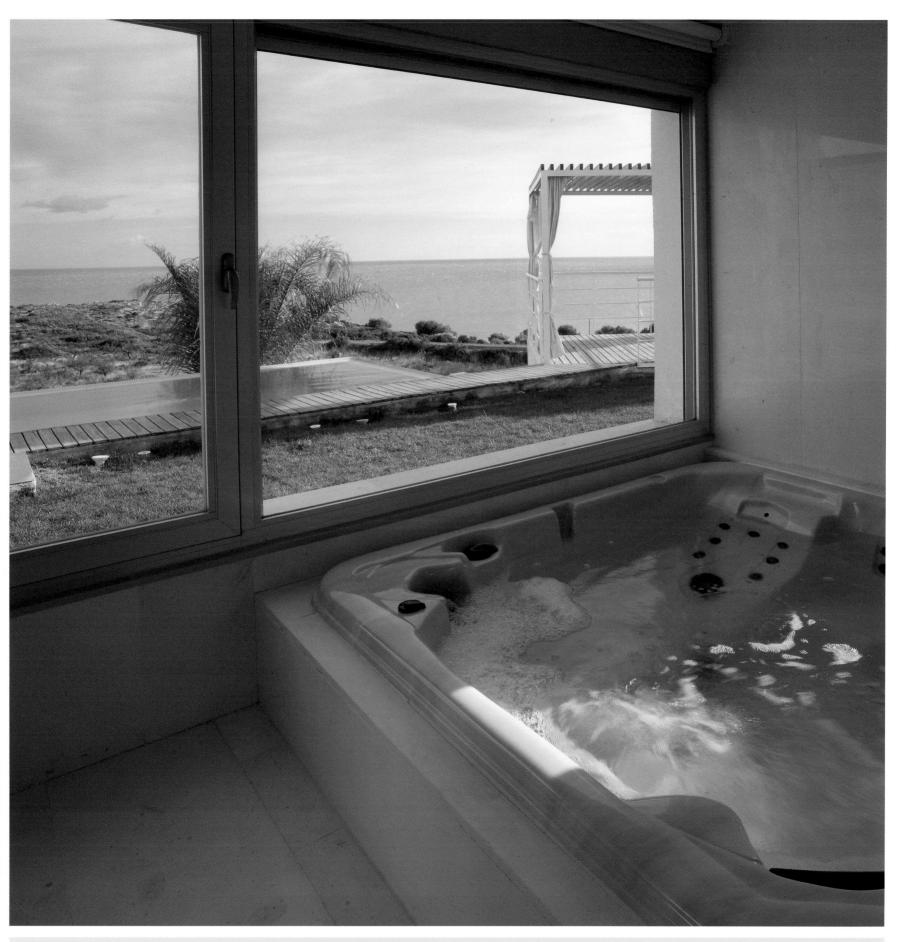

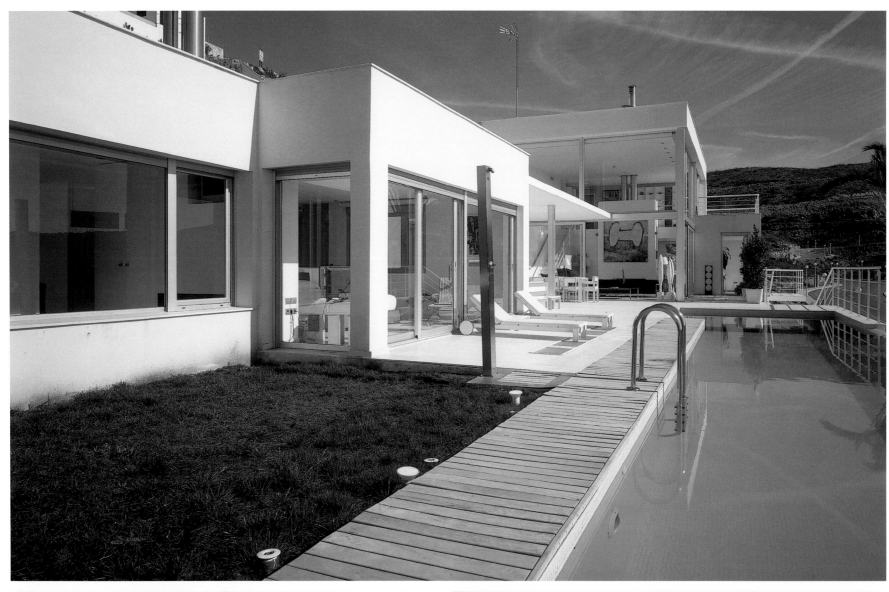

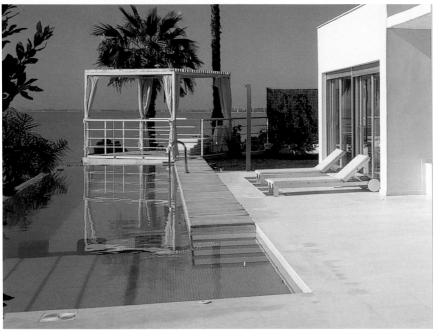

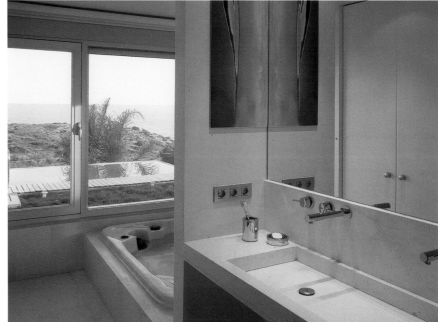

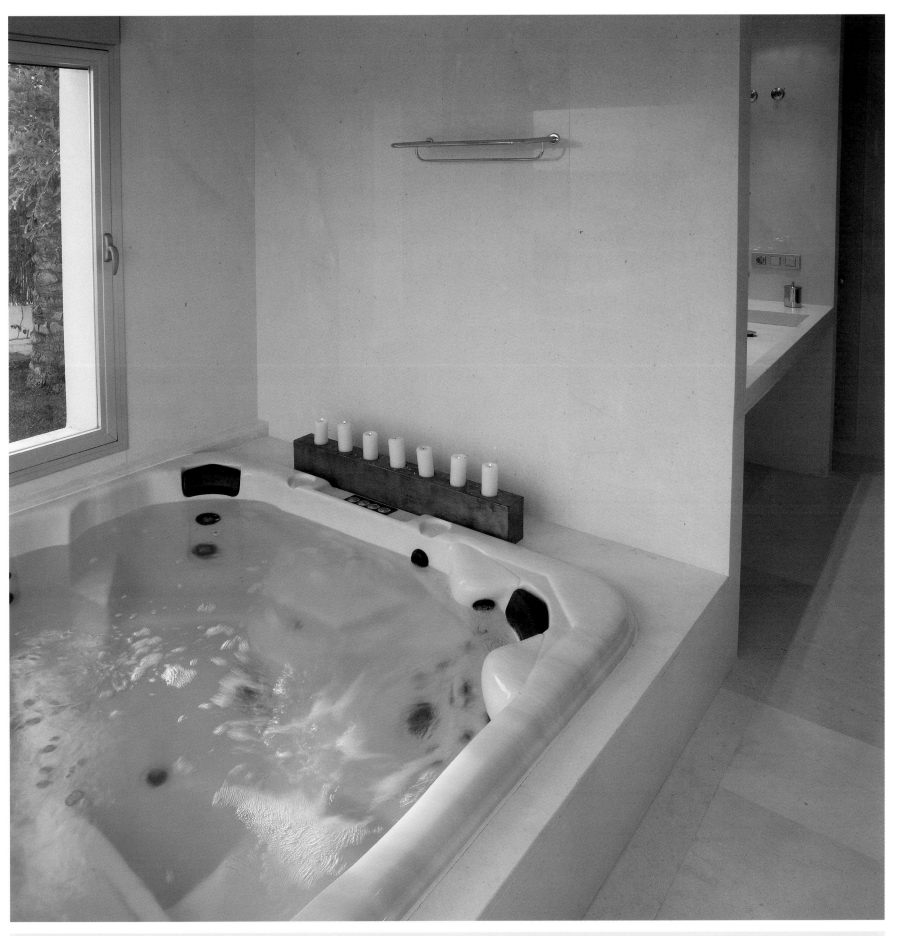

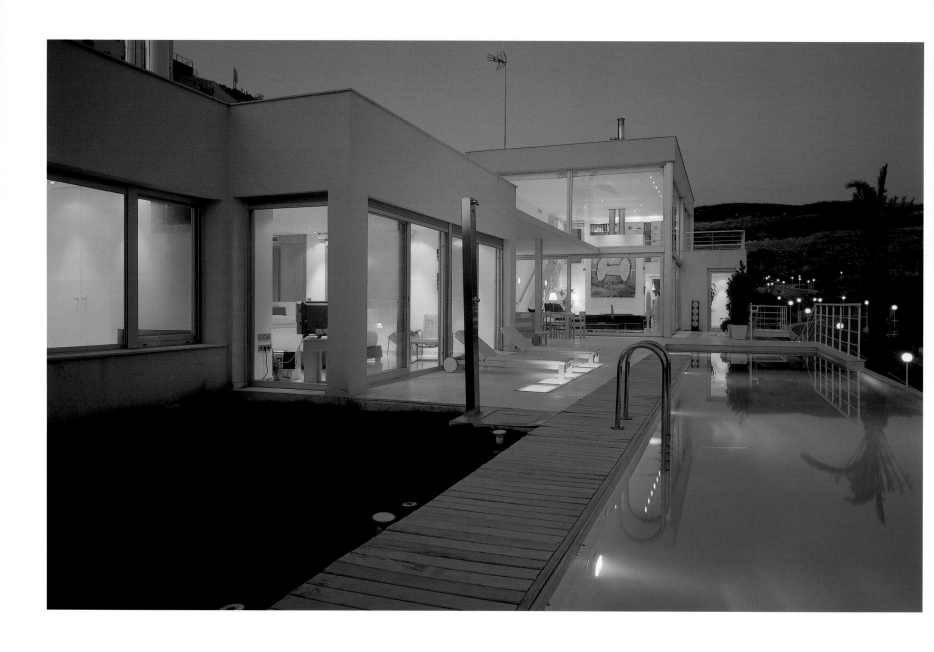

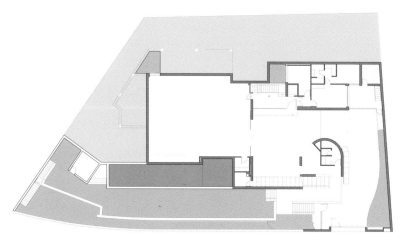

Plan

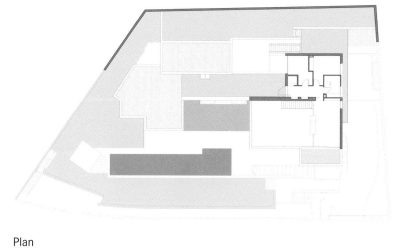

Plan

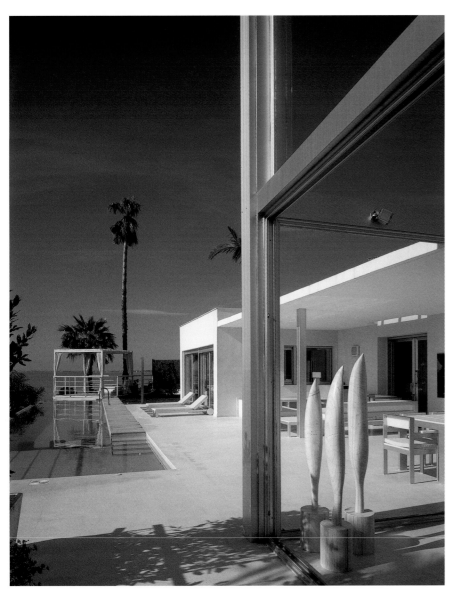

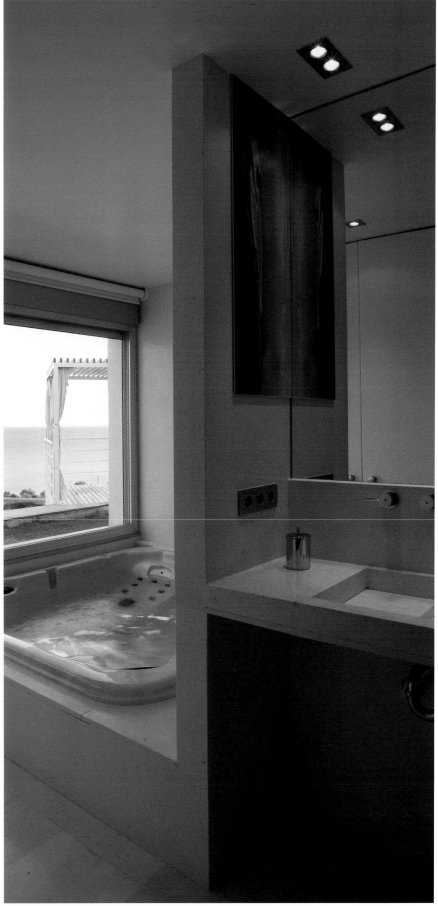

The design of the bathroom fuses conventional features with those of the most lavish of spas: the shower doubles as a steam bath and the bathtub also offers a hydromassage.

A Residence on Old Branchville Road

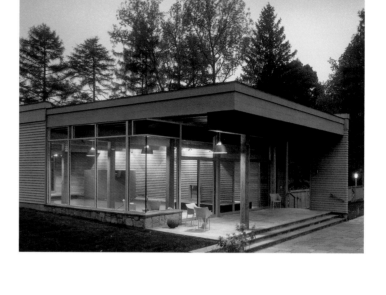

The covered pool is one of the most important elements in the enlargement of this home. It comprises a structure that is completely made out of wood and whose cedar beams reflect the solidity of this high-ceiling residence. The skylights and the large proportion of glazed façade offer striking views of the forest that surrounds the dwelling. The pool extends out from a low wall, out of which flows a cascade of water; on the opposite end, a square bath offers one the opportunity to enjoy a hydromassage. The wall, bath, and pool are clad in blue glass tiles, in stark contrast to the intense green of the surrounding vegetation. Simple, straight lines and high-quality materials round out this luxuriously finished house, in which one can enjoy a swim or a hydromassage any time of year.

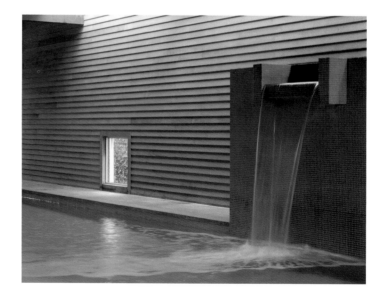

Architect: **Donald Billinkoff Architects**
Location: **Ridgefield, Connecticut, United States**
Photos © **Donald Martinez, Mark Samu and**
 Elliot Kaufman

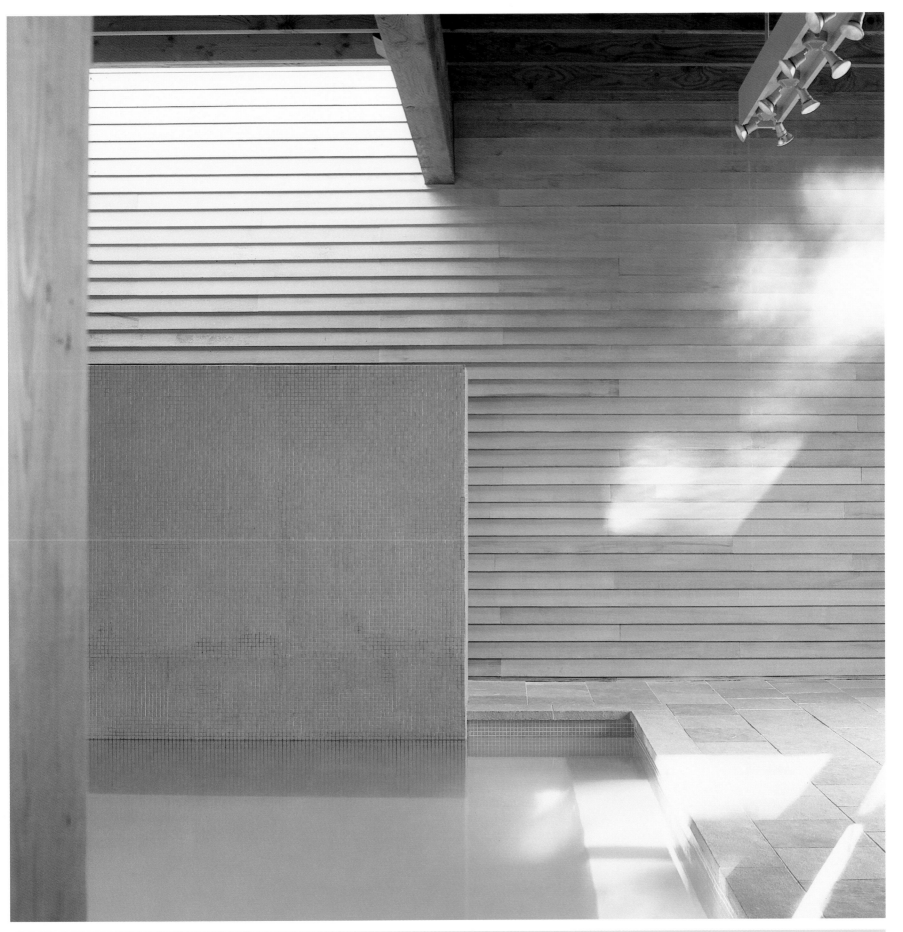

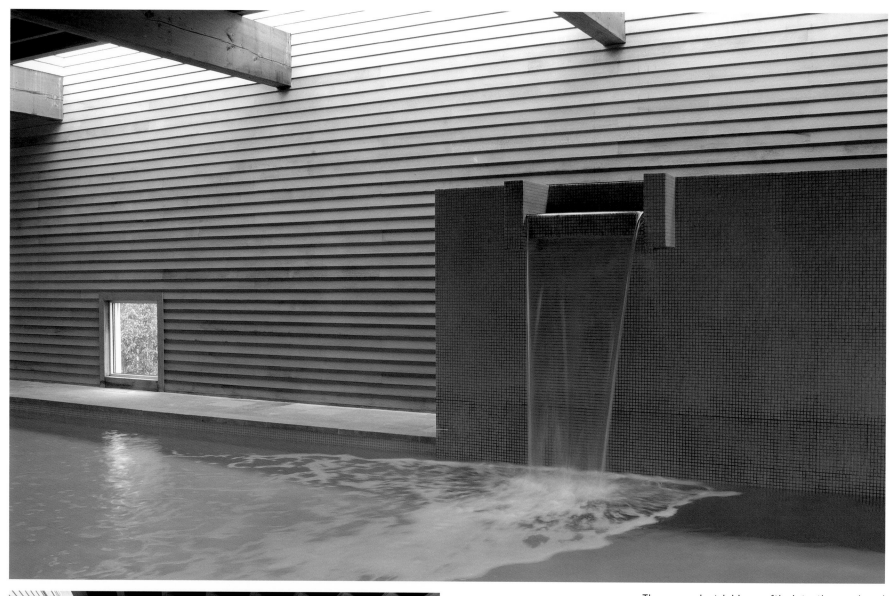

The cascade trickles softly into the pool and renews a constant, cyclical movement of water that brings this place to life.

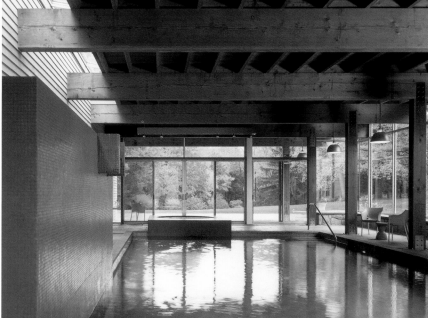

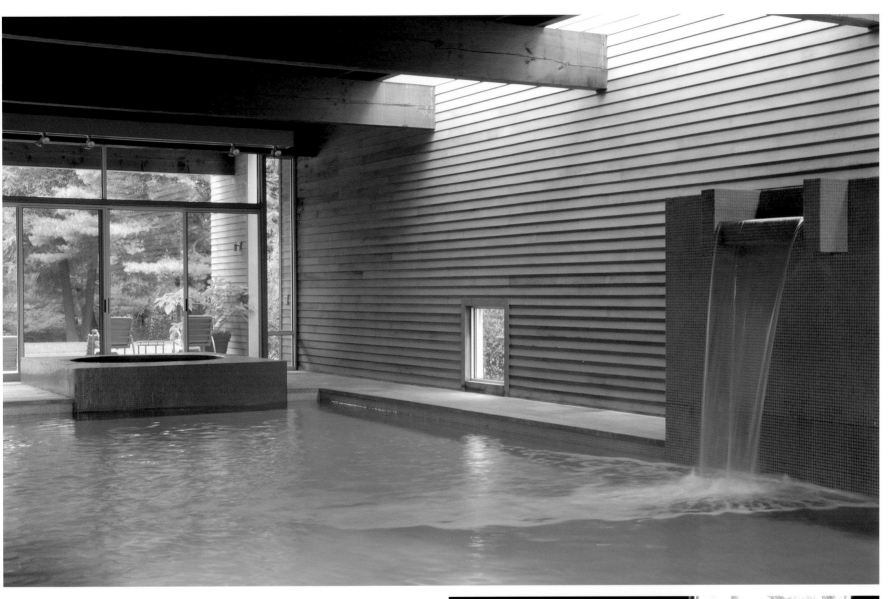

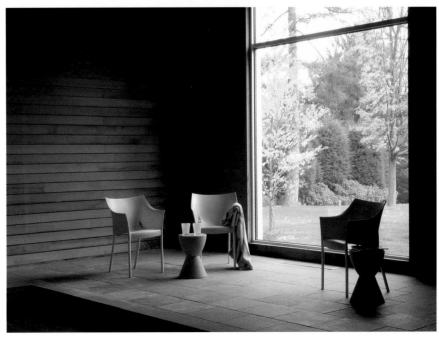

Ofuro

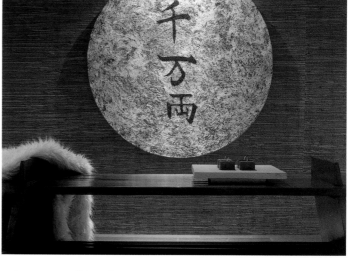

Japanese tradition dictates the custom of the *ofuro*, in which people gather every day in a room dedicated to relaxation. This deeply rooted practice entails a hot-water bath—at a temperature between 104 and 107.6 °F—whose function is not to clean, but rather to eliminate toxins, relax one's muscles, stimulate relaxation, and purify both body and soul. Recent interest in everything Eastern has brought it to the West. *Ofuro* is a bath that does not require soap, mineral salts, or any other aromatic substance, as the bathtubs themselves were traditionally crafted from hinoki, a fragrant wood whose aromas impregnated the steam coming off the hot water. This project, then, is a combination of high-quality materials and a Japanese aesthetic: the floor is paved in ipé wood, slate covers the walls, and tatami mats are spread across the living-room floor. These materials combine to create a relaxing atmosphere, which is counteracted by the technology that maintains the temperature of the bath at 107.6 °F— which guarantees that bathers' well-being will be enhanced.

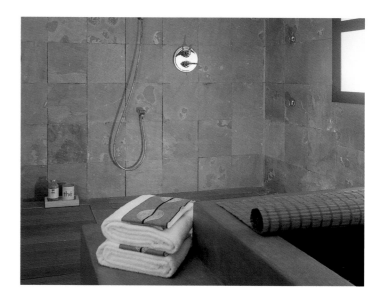

Interior Design: **Bárbara Sindreu/CAD Interiorismo**
Location: **Barcelona, Spain**
Photos © **Núria Fuentes**

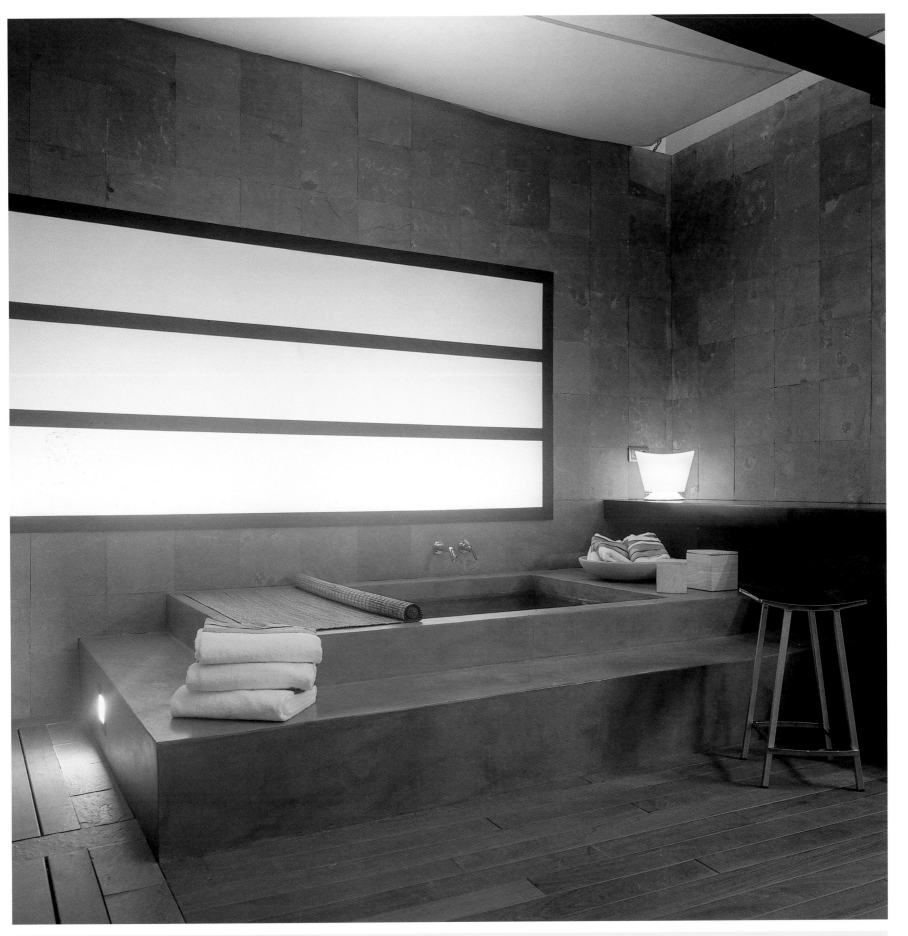

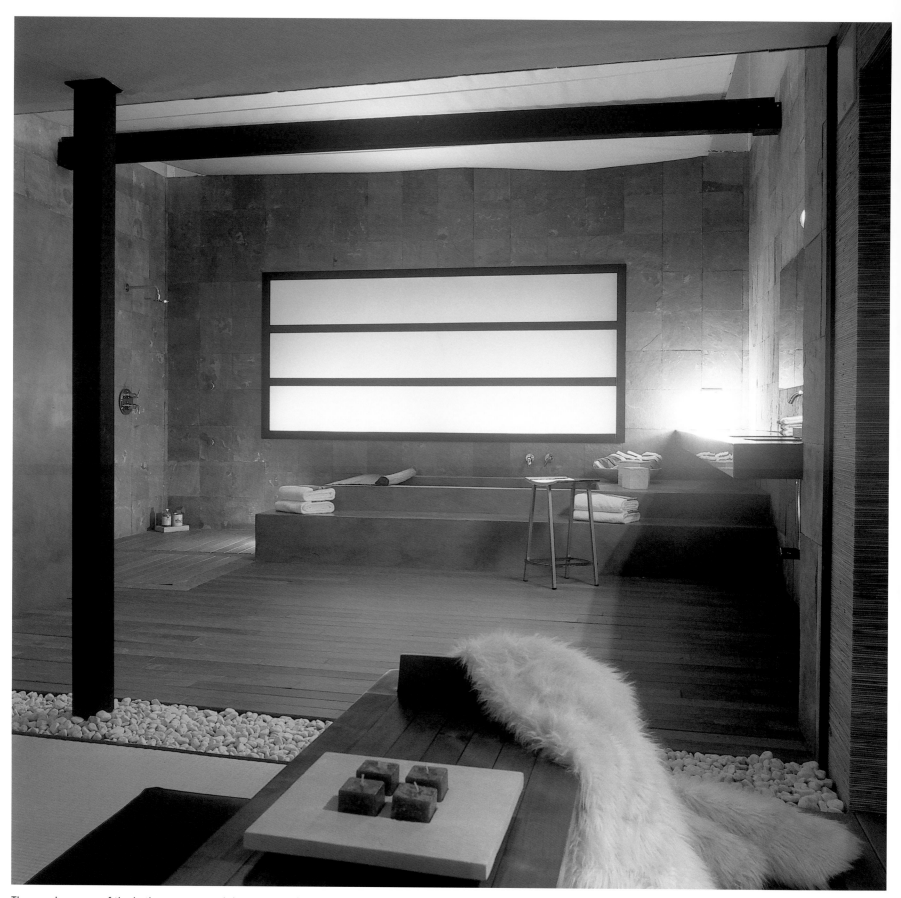

The spaciousness of the bathroom area and the austere décor yield a serene and placid atmosphere in which one can disconnect from the outside world and purify one's body.

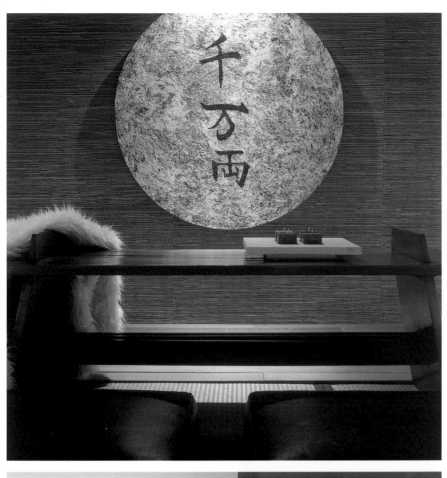

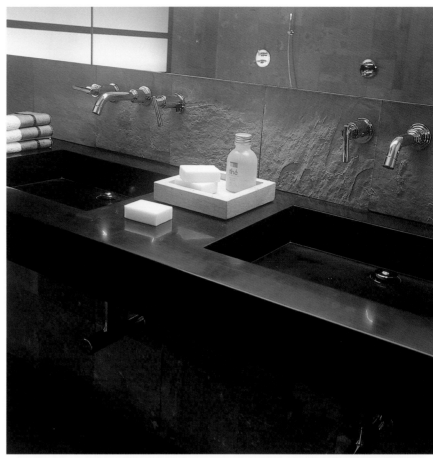

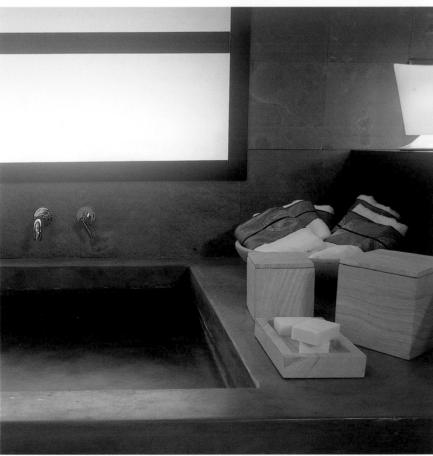

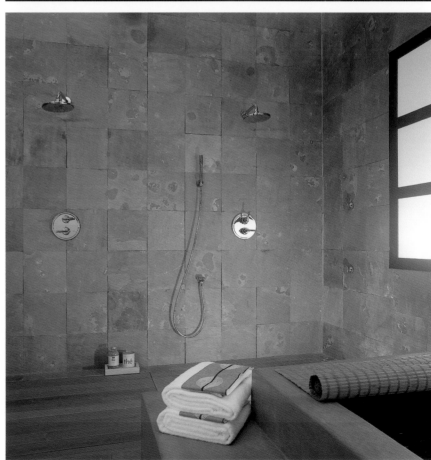

Levallois Pool

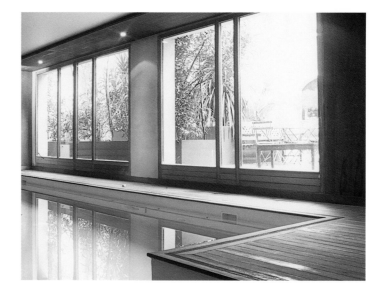

The main objective behind this project was to install a covered pool, a gym, and a sauna in a space that had previously been occupied by the garage of a house. This change in how this space was to be used clearly reflects the vitality of the client: a space that had previously been reserved for cars was converted into a spacious area dedicated to exercise, health, and well-being. Natural materials, such as stone and wood, were chosen for this transformation, as they symbolize solidity, depth, and transparency. Water and light were also given precedence in the search for a warm and natural ambience. The glass wall allows the greens of the foliage on the terrace to penetrate into the interior, which is itself bathed in blue. In keeping with the Latin maxim *mens sana in corpore sano*, the sauna, which is located in a quieter and more intimate spot, offers a place for relaxing and purifying the body after a workout.

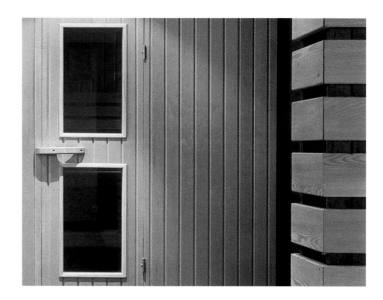

Architect: **Guilhem Roustan**
Location: **Île-de-France, France**
Photos © **Daniel Moulinet**

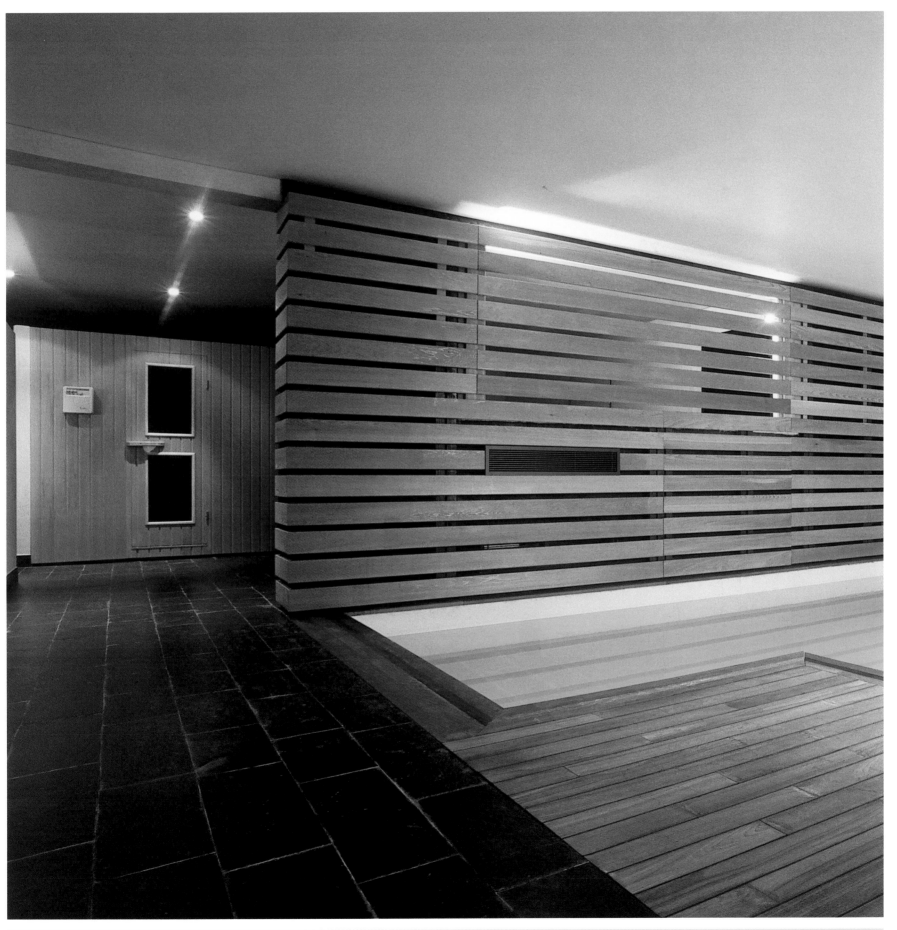

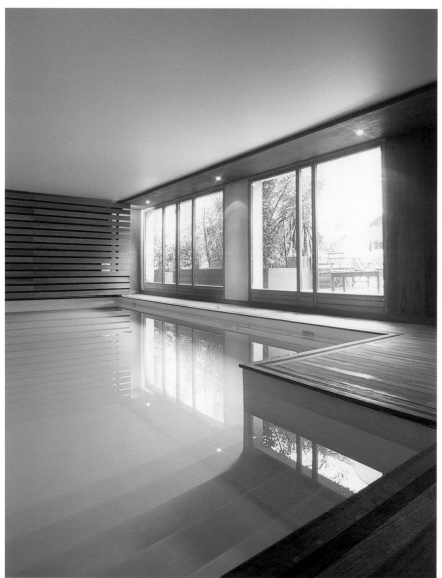

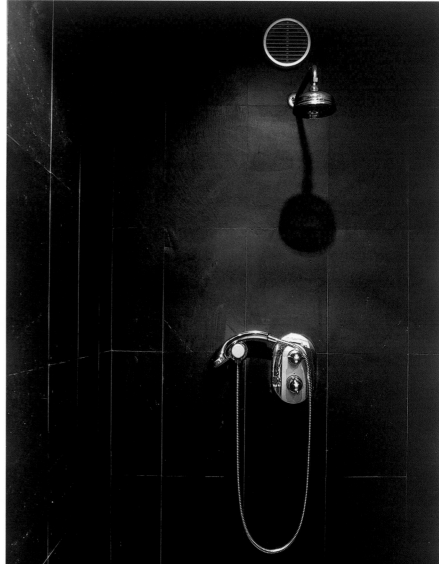

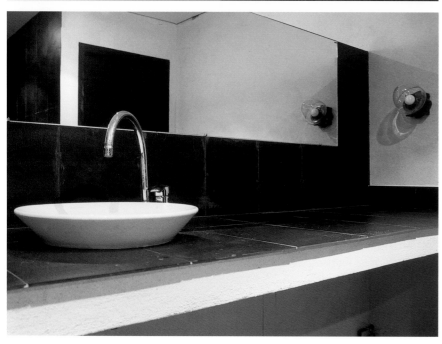

The wood on the walls in the pool area creates a warm atmosphere that contrasts with the darker color of the tiles.

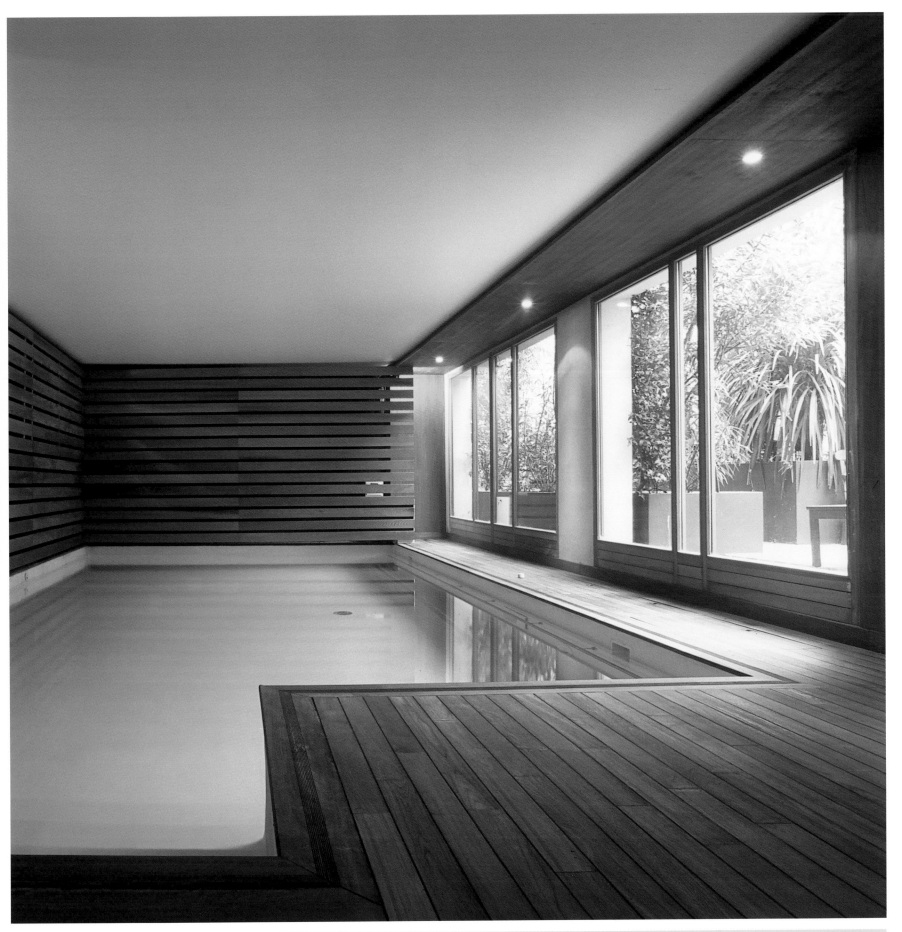

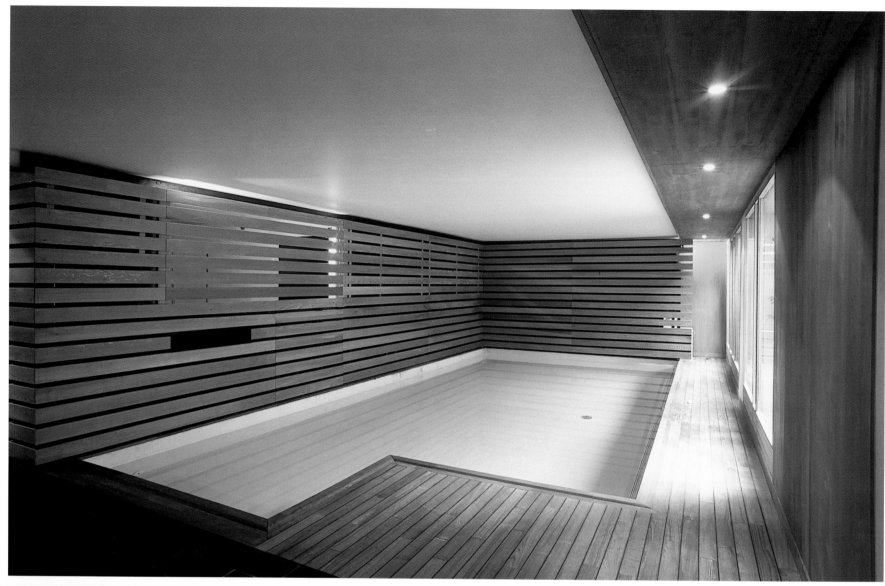

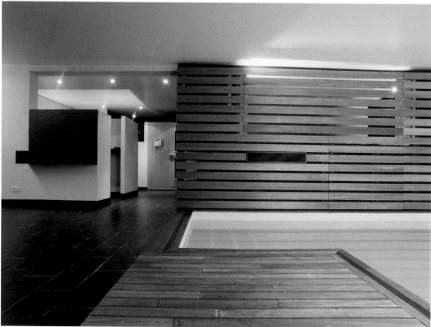

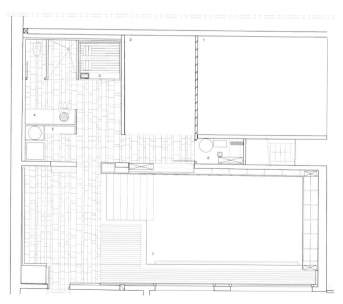

Plan

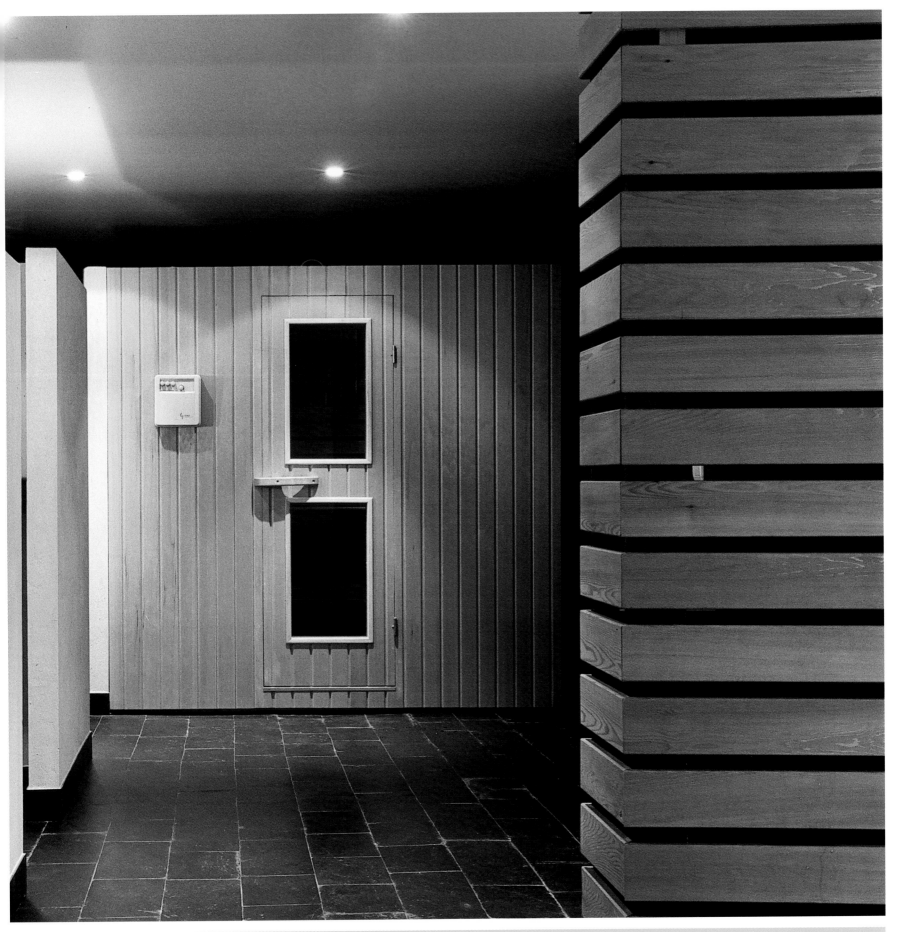

A Penthouse in Valencia

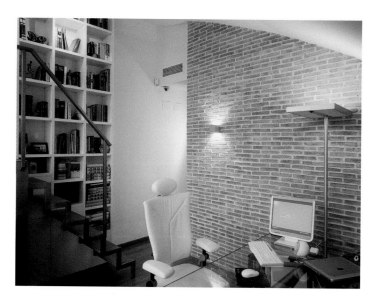

This exceptional two-story house enjoys views out over the sea, the port, and the fertile lands around Valencia, and is furthermore completely open to the exterior, thanks to a large, glazed façade. The spacious terraces, one of which is closed, provide space in which to rest. The upper level of the duplex is located beneath a vaulted ceiling, which came to determine how the spaces would be distributed. The main bedroom includes a light-filled hydromassage bath, which is located under the highest point of the vault: the bath is thus rendered the most important element in the room. These two functions—that of bathroom and that of bedroom—are separated by a transparent glass screen. The privileged location of the bath means that it dominates the entire space in such a way that its presence is a constant reminder of the possibility of taking a relaxing bath. The wood floors, along with the décor, give rise to a welcoming suite, and the large windows take advantage of the light of the Mediterranean to fill the room with energy.

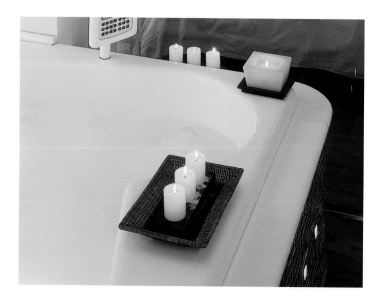

Architect: **Jorge Segarra**
Location: **Valencia, Spain**
Photos © **Joan Roig**

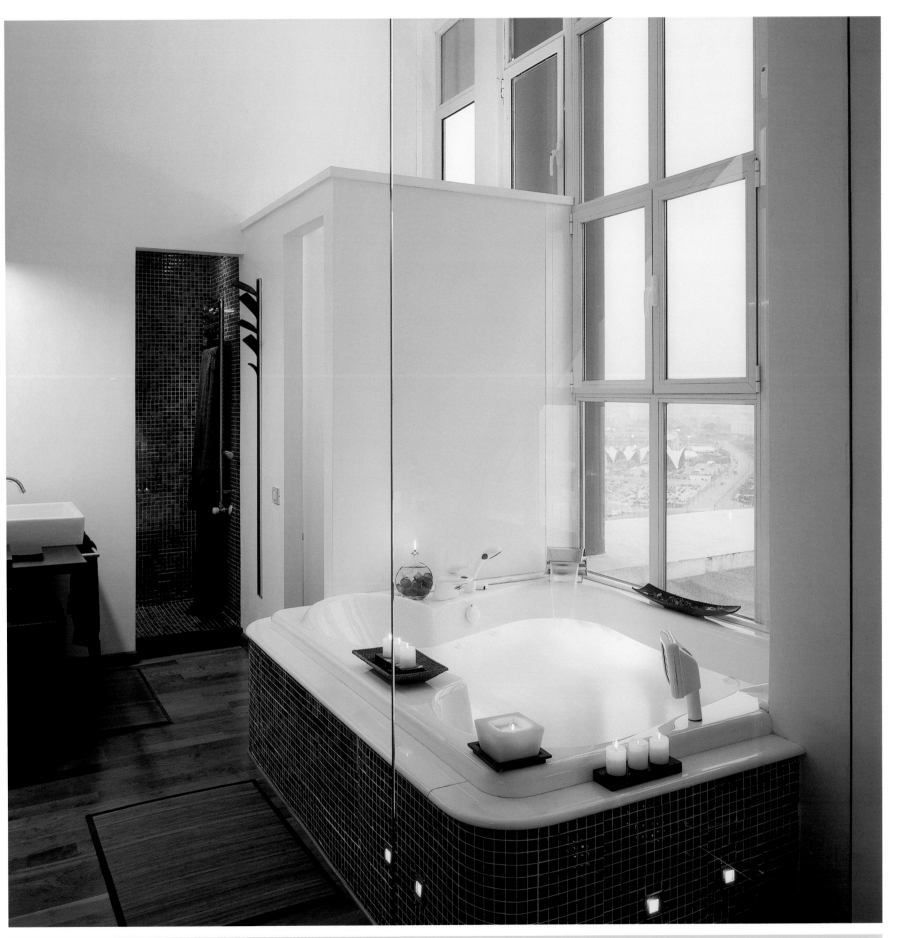

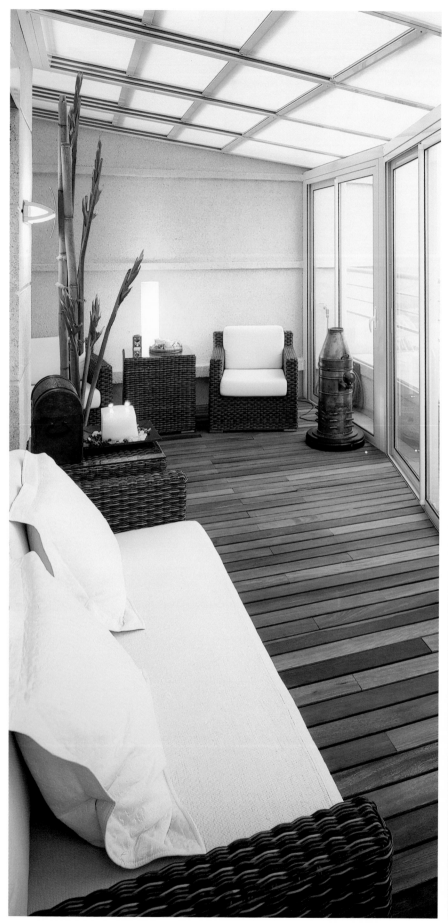

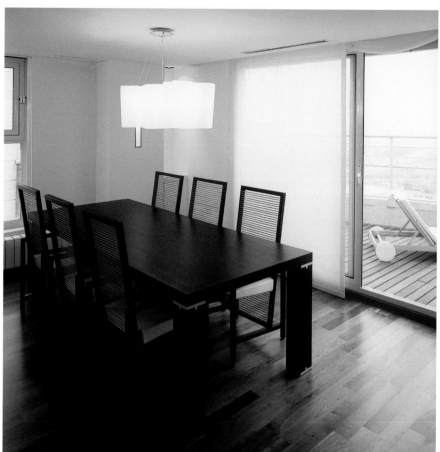

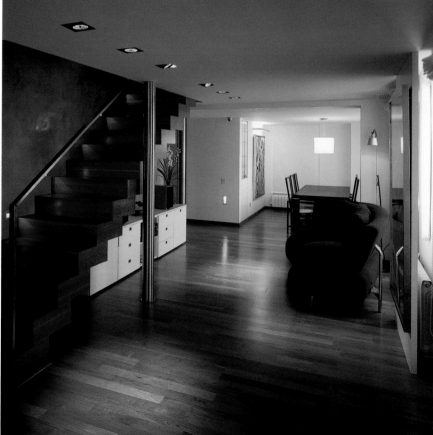

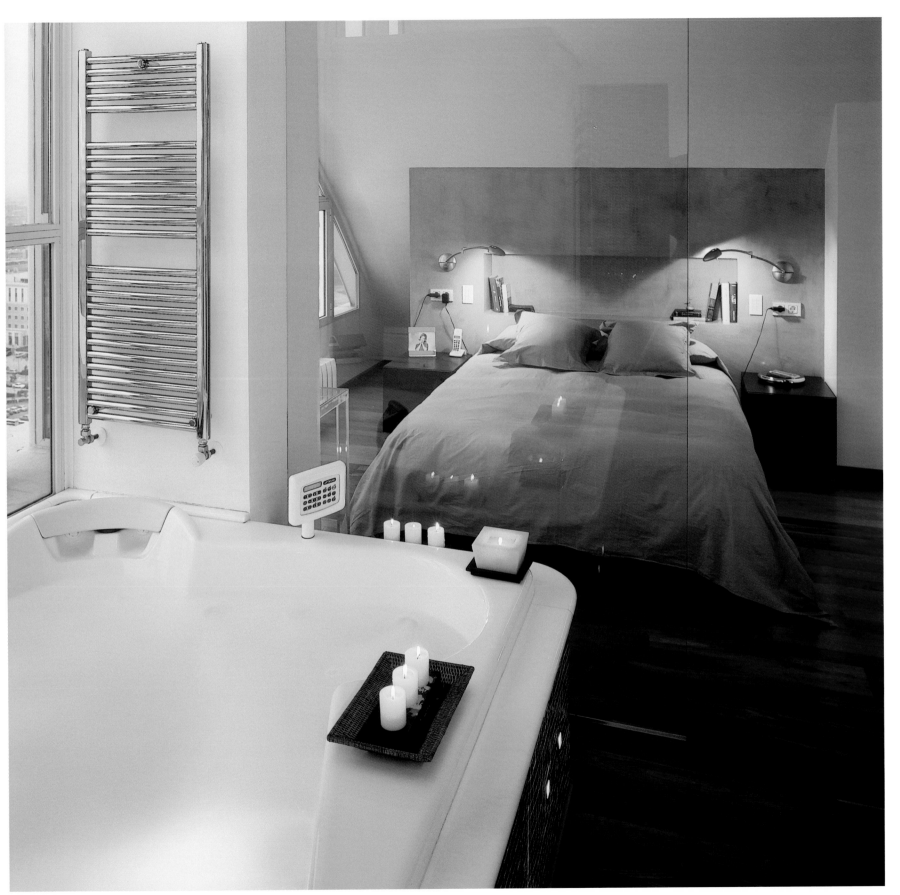

The bedroom and the bathroom are separated by a glass screen that creates a division that is more conceptual than visual.

A House on Monte Tauro

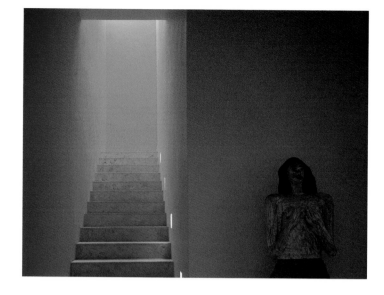

This house was designed as a refuge from the chaos of the big city. As an example of the idea the architects were after, a central, open-air space creates an atmosphere for resting, reading, and conversation, while remaining fully private. A narrow staircase leads to the bedroom, bathroom, and gym, the latter of which has a sliding glass ceiling that lets natural light and air in whenever one chooses. The luminosity and bright colors are the two things that best personify this dwelling—this is especially seen in the gym, where the salmon-colored walls create an air of vitality and energy. A small pool lets one relax and cool off while enjoying the views of the landscape that surrounds the house. A bathroom and shower round out the simple and elegant forms of this small temple to relaxation.

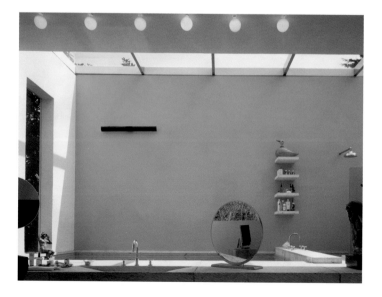

Architect: **Legorreta y Legorreta**
Location: **Mexico City, Mexico**
Photos © **Lourdes Legorreta**

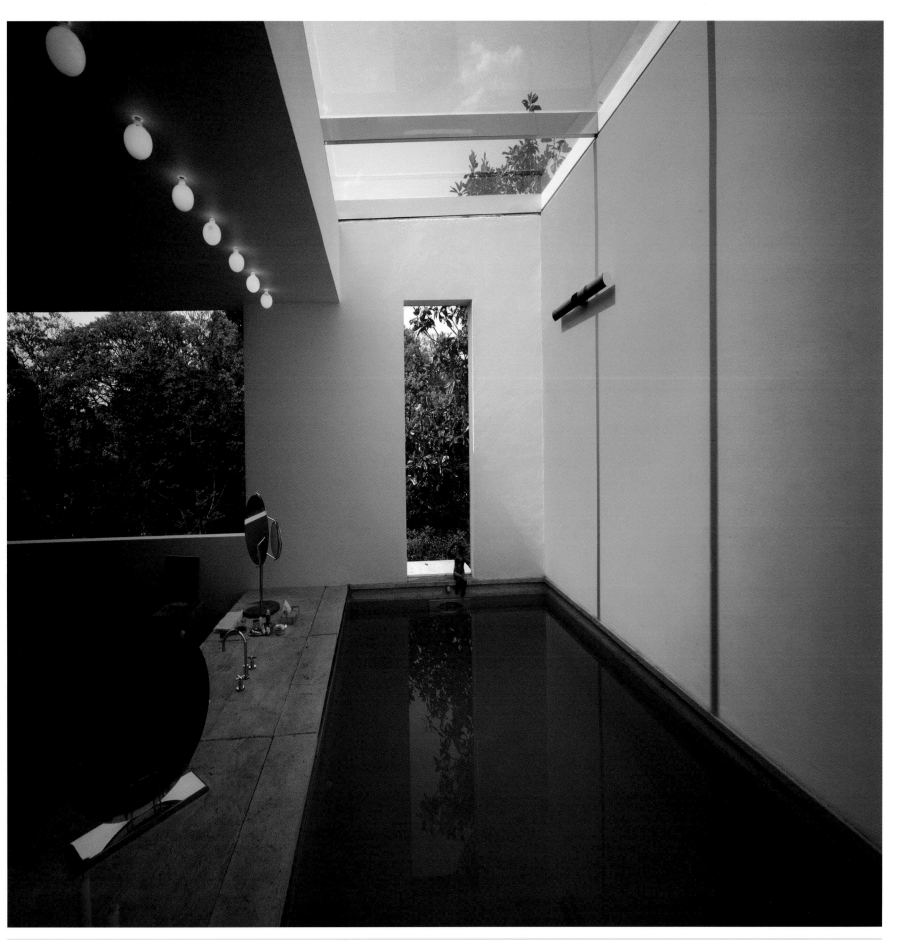

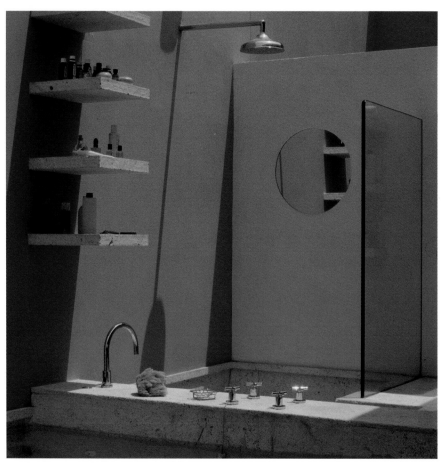
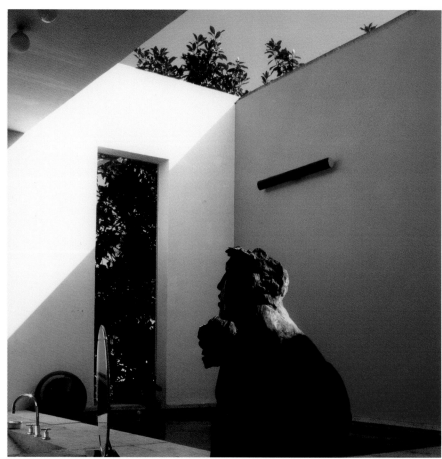

Luminosity and color are two characteristics of this spa; natural light floods the interior and rose-colored tones lend vitality.

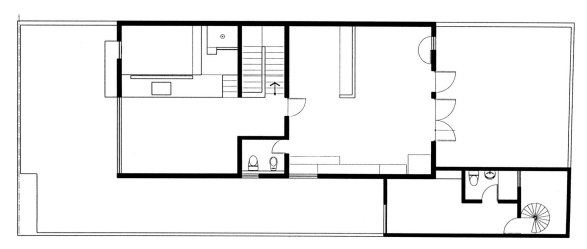

Plan

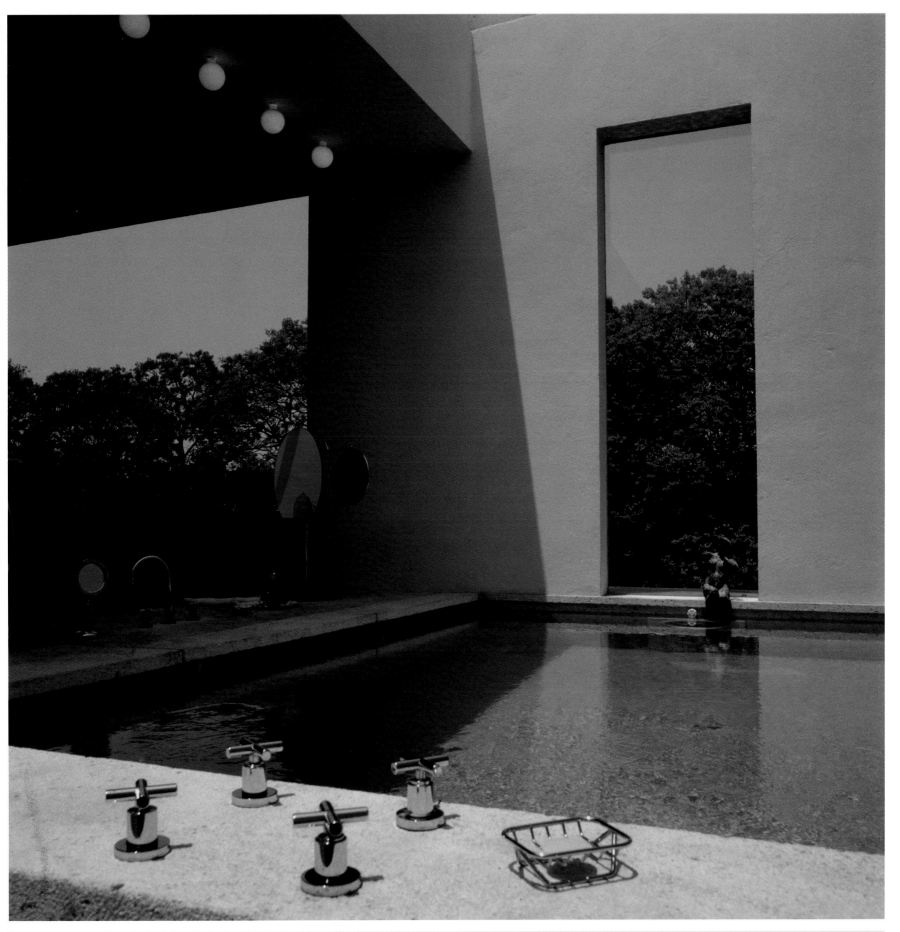

Slefringe Residence

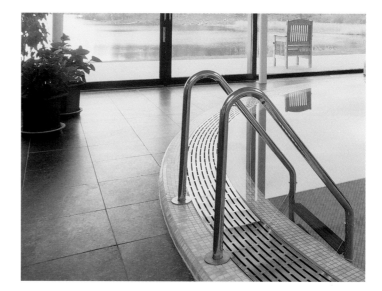

The aim of the most recent renovation of this house was to install a spa, which houses a covered pool, sauna, shower, and bar in a covered building oriented—via a glass façade—toward the adjacent lake. The pool is elliptical in shape and the water surface is slightly above ground level, which gives one the sensation of swimming in the lake when really in the pool. An ellipsoid volume contains the sauna, from which one can also contemplate the lake, thanks to a window that opens onto the glass façade. Another unique volume, in which two halves of a cylinder form an S shape, houses the shower and bar. Both the pool and the volumes are clad in tesseras of mosaic tile in a range of different shades of blue. The Norwegian granite of the floor extends all the way out to the terrace to establish continuity with the interior; this continuity is even more evident in summer, when the large windows are left open.

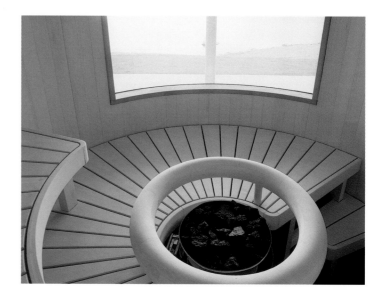

Architect: **Mikael Bergquist Arkitektkontor**
Location: **Östergötland, Sweden**
Photos © **James Silverman**

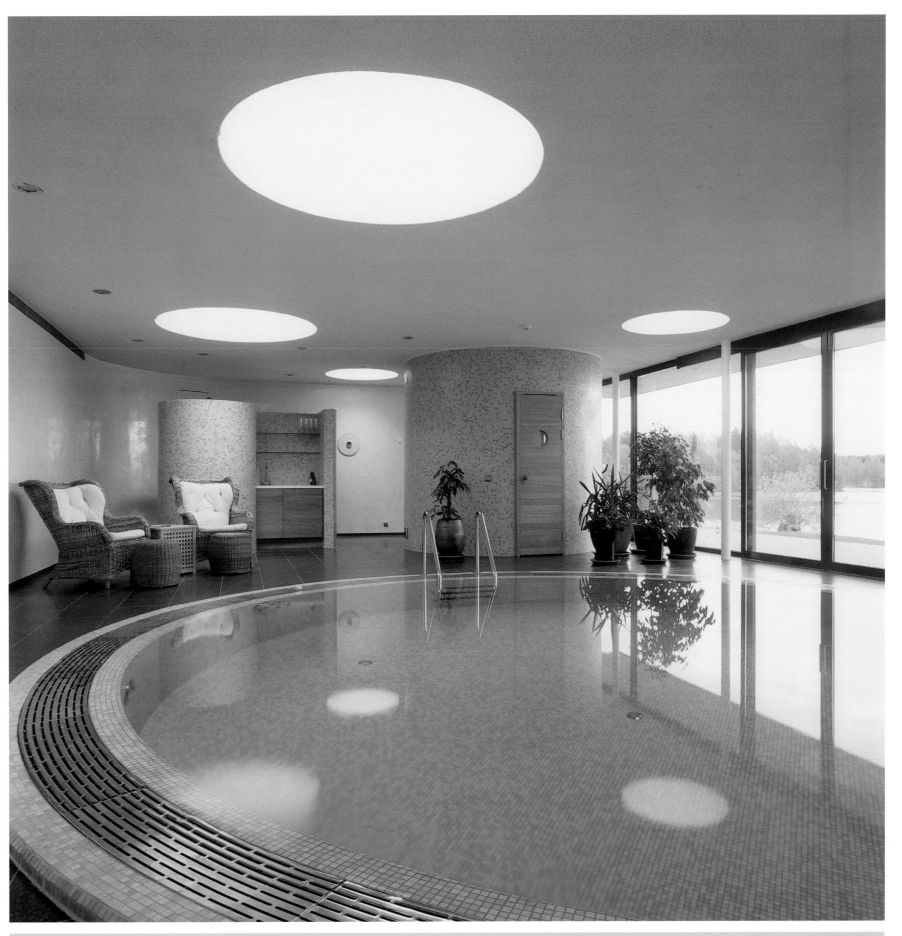

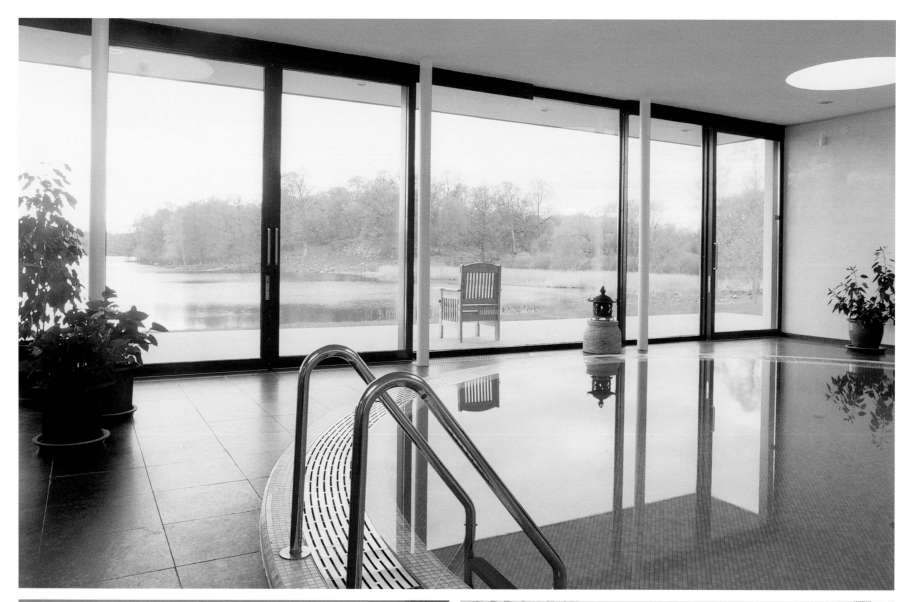

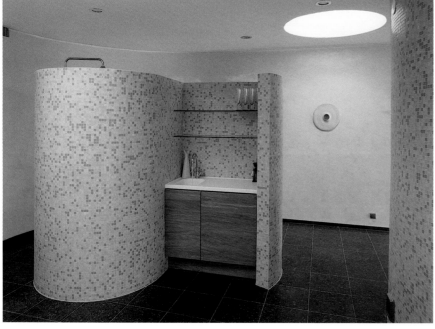

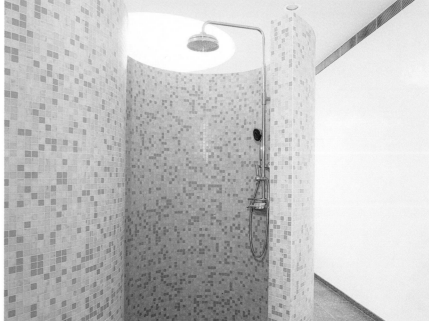

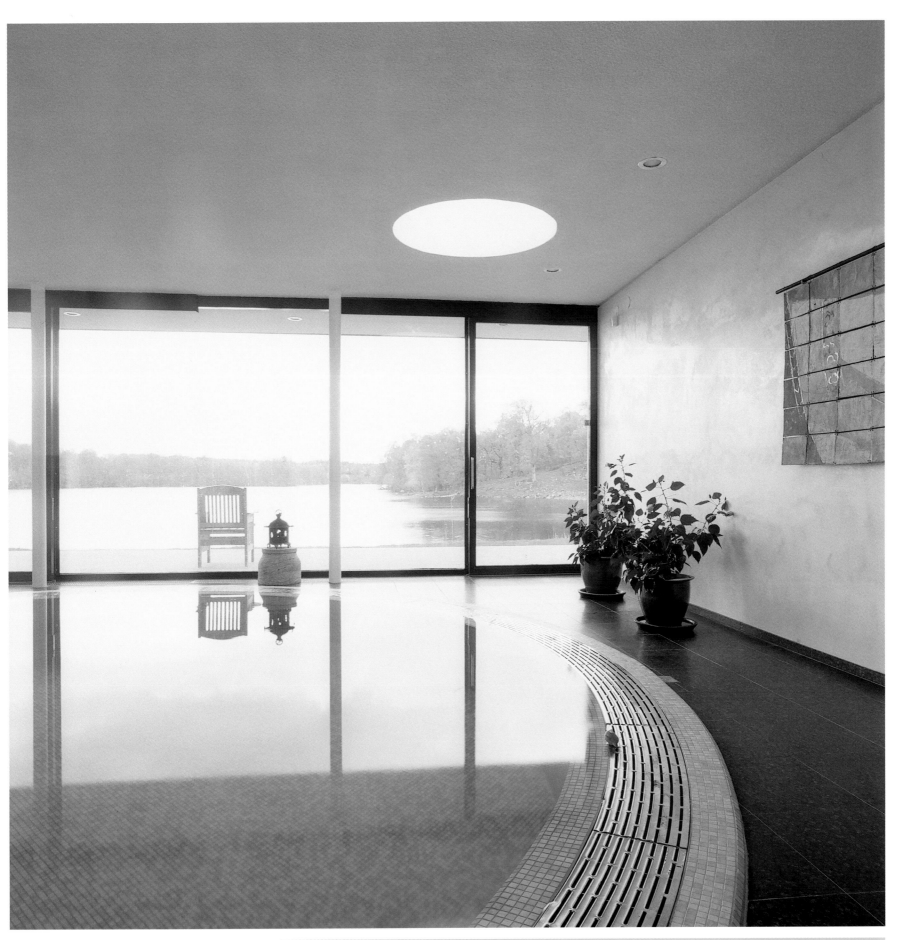

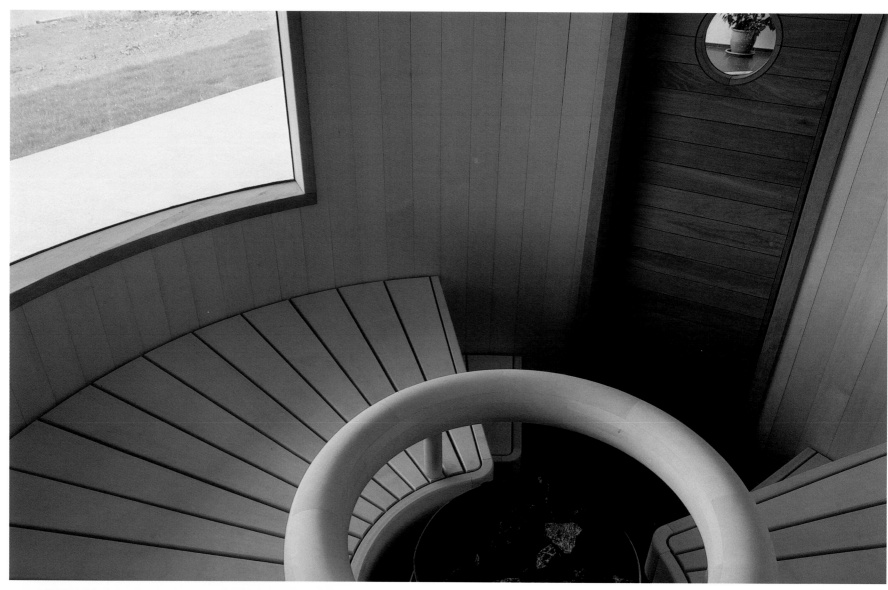

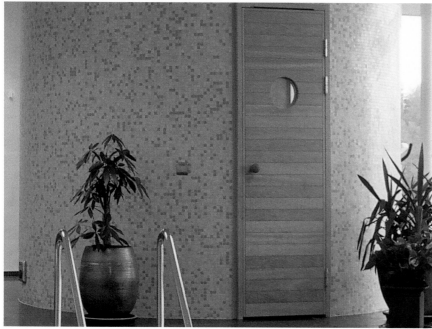

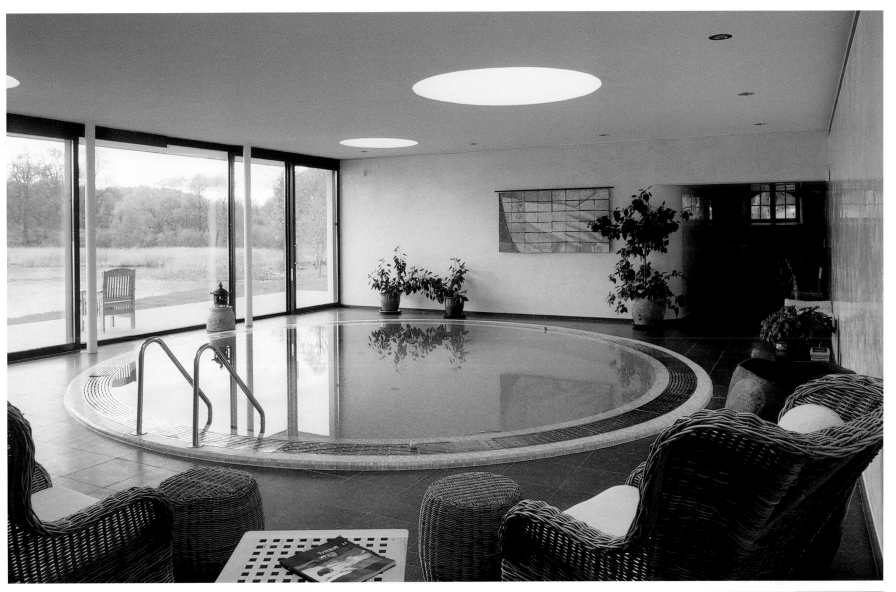

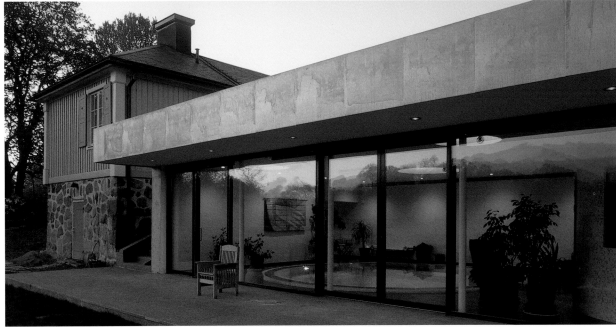

One can enjoy this spa during any season of the year: in winter it is closed off from the outside and in summer the glass walls can be opened to take advantage of good weather.

A Villa
in Gordes

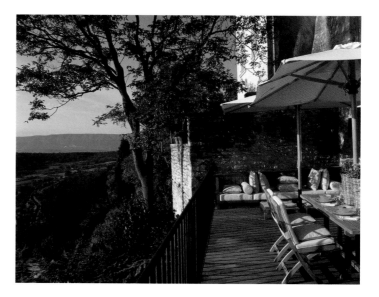

The medieval village of Gordes, in Provence, was chosen by this decorator and designer for her weekend residence. The objective was to achieve a place that would serve as a source of inspiration and contemplation and would be far from the hustle and bustle of Paris. The entire house was thus designed by the owner herself, who was inspired by Asian culture. The sensitivity of Zen Buddhism or feng shui is reflected in the furniture and the arrangement of all the elements in the house. In the small pool and bathing area, which is located in what once served as a stable, one can bask in an ambience of relaxation and quiet. The stone arch and Carrara marble define a natural space that evokes the baths of ancient Rome, as though the space were a *caldarium* or *frigidarium*. The harmony of lines and purity of materials define a corner for enjoying the tranquility and silence to which one can escape from the big city.

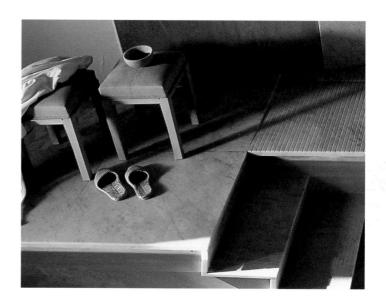

Architect: **Lilia Konrad/LKD Concepts**
Location: **Gordes, France**
Photos © **Reto Guntli/Zapaimages**

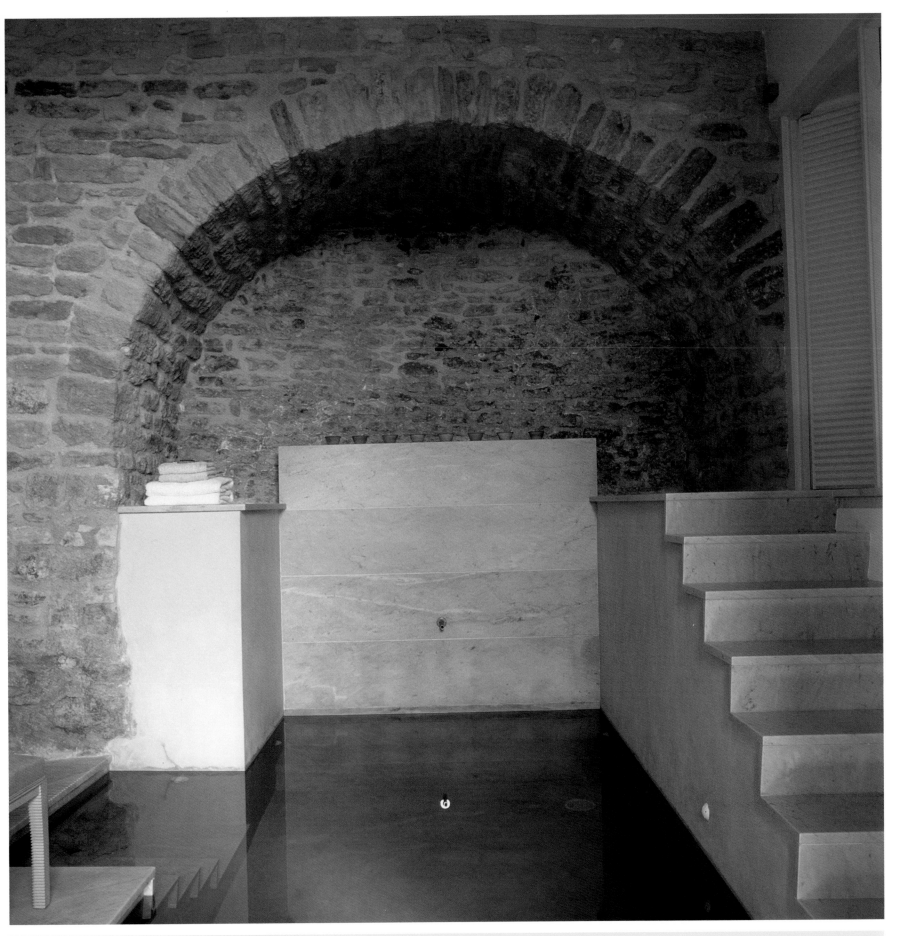

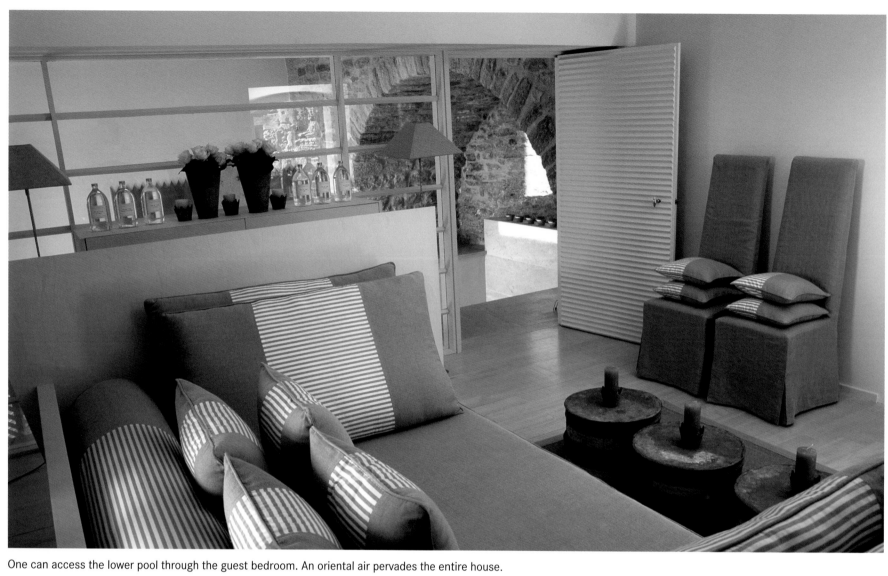

One can access the lower pool through the guest bedroom. An oriental air pervades the entire house.

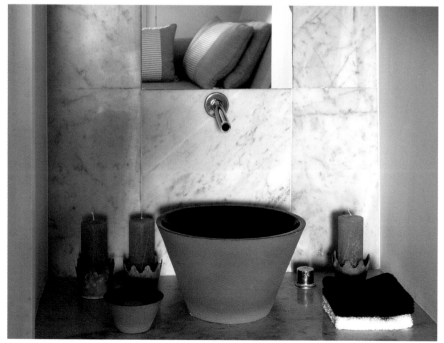

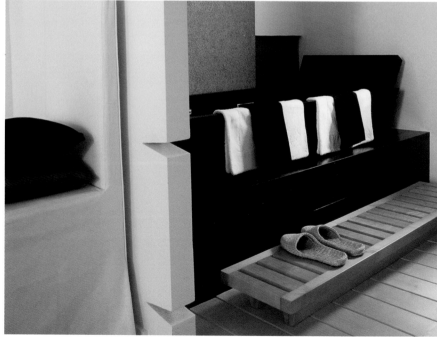

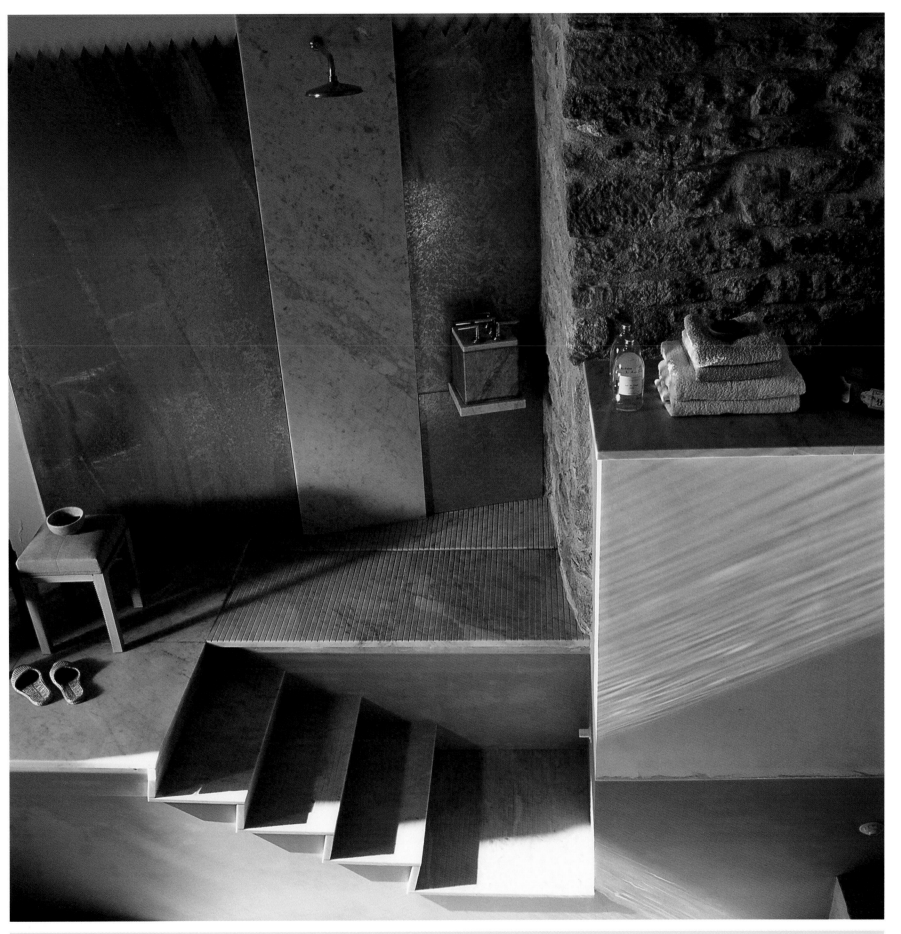

Hilltop Residence

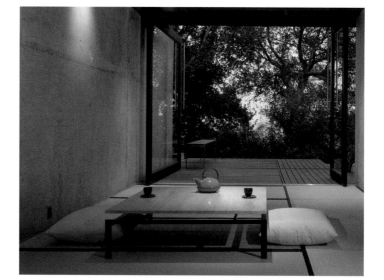

This house, designed in the 1950s by architect Thornton Ladd, enjoys spectacular views of Pasadena, the San Fernando Valley, and the surrounding mountains. The architects chosen to renovate it maintained the original relationship between interior and exterior, and sought to bring out vertical and horizontal planes throughout. The Asian influences on the owner's tastes are evident in both the architecture and the decoration, and are reflected more succinctly in the bedroom and the ofuro, or Japanese bath. According to Japanese tradition, hot water contained in a wooden tub helps to boost one's mental and spiritual well-being, and the shower with hydromassage represents the modern addition to this very complete spa. By varying the pressure and temperature of the water in the shower, one can invigorate the muscles and stimulate blood flow. The natural landscape surrounding the house is the perfect environment for finding peace and relaxation and escaping from one's everyday obligations.

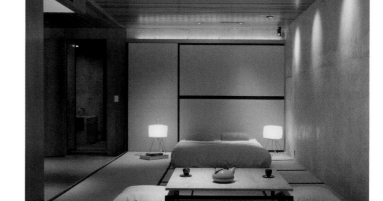

Architect: **Marmol Radziner and Associates**
Location: **Pasadena, California, United States**
Photos © **Benny Chan/Fotoworks**

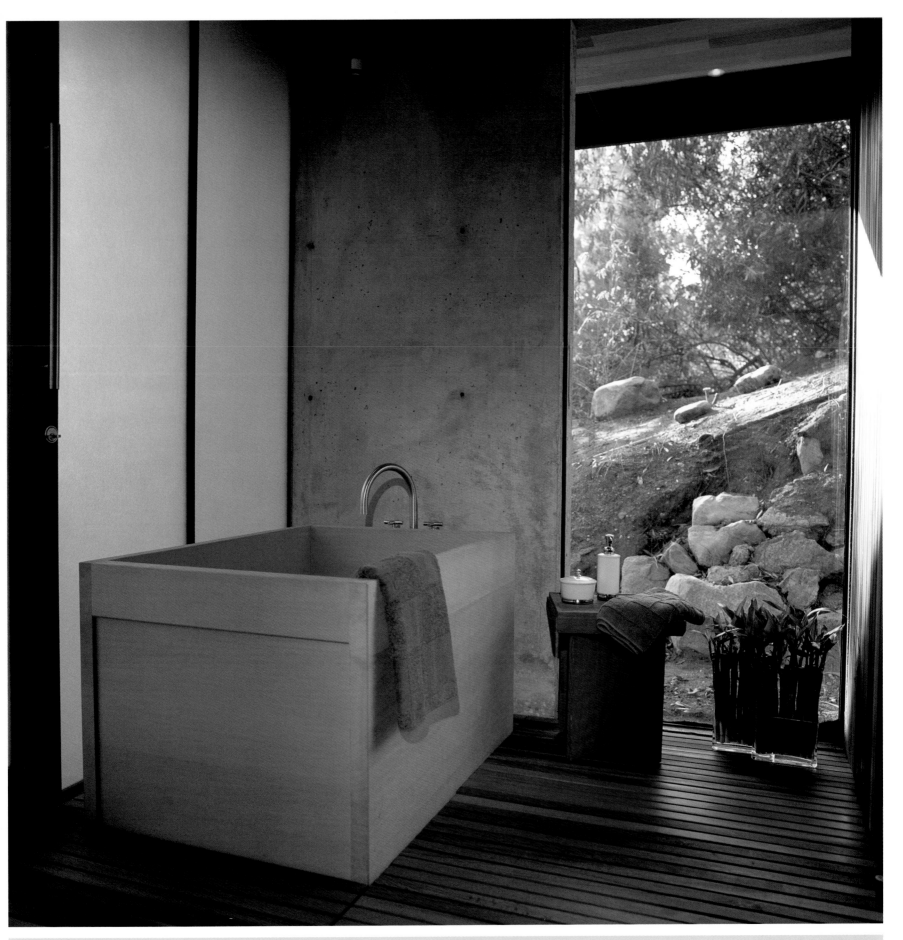

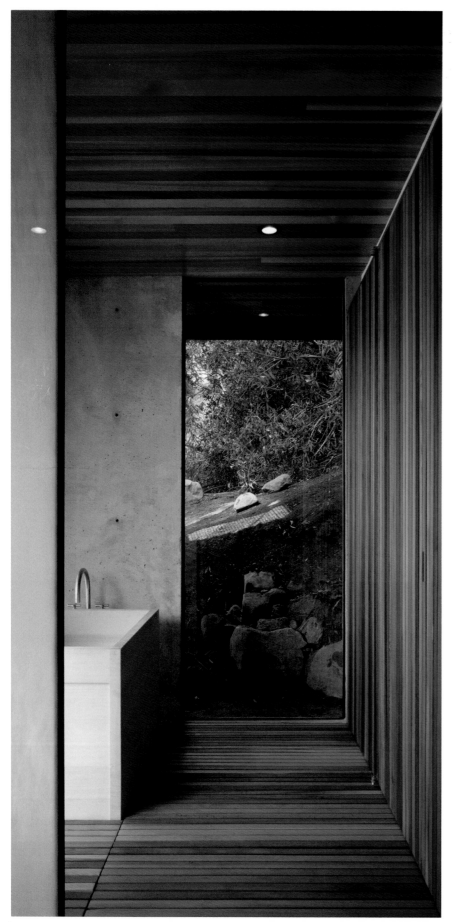

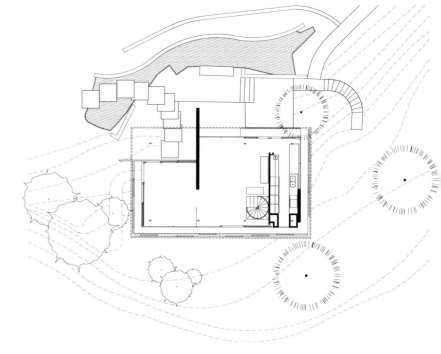

Upper level

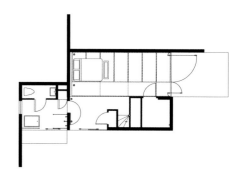

Lower level

Wood, which is used throughout the bathroom, provides a warm and comforting atmosphere. The views to the outside accentuate the relationship between architecture and nature.

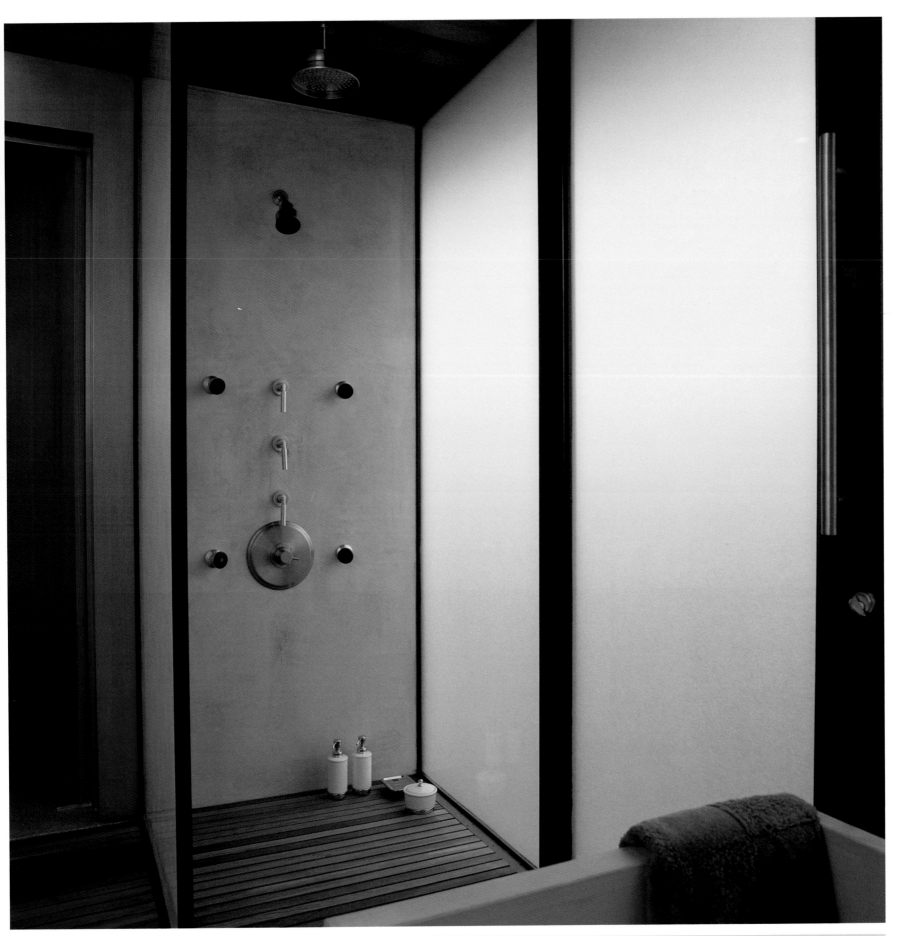

Espacio Wellness

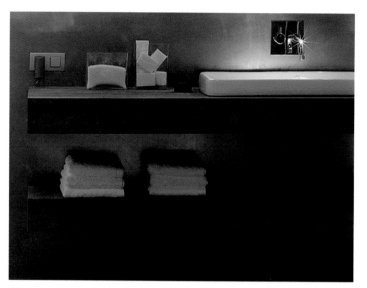

Over the years, bathrooms have moved from the sidelines to center stage in houses, which has led to more innovative designs and ever more sophisticated offerings. This project, which entailed the design of a bath whose aesthetic would be both youthful and industrial in inspiration, was to be fitted into a loft-style space that would be open and spacious and benefit from high ceilings and the latest in designer furniture. In addition to the typical elements found in baths, it also includes showers, wall bars, and a sauna, all of which are manufactured by Ideal Standard. As the concept of wellness combines exercise, toning, and relaxation, this spa functions as either a gym, a place for relaxation, or a traditional bathhouse, all of which can be performed in a series of comfortable, purpose-driven spaces. The steel-plated walls serve a double function: they both conceal the services and facilities and lend privacy to the spaces. Waterproof sucupira wood provides the touch of warmth needed to transform this space into a comfortable and elegant place in which to reestablish the equilibrium between body and mind.

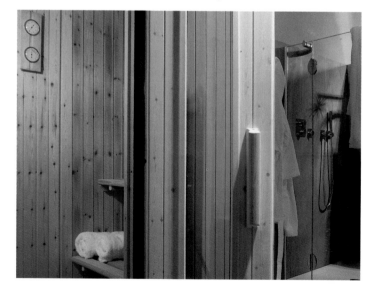

Architect/Interior Designer: **Anna Generó/Ivalo**
Location: **Barcelona, Spain**
Photos © **Núria Fuentes, Ideal Standard**

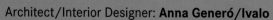

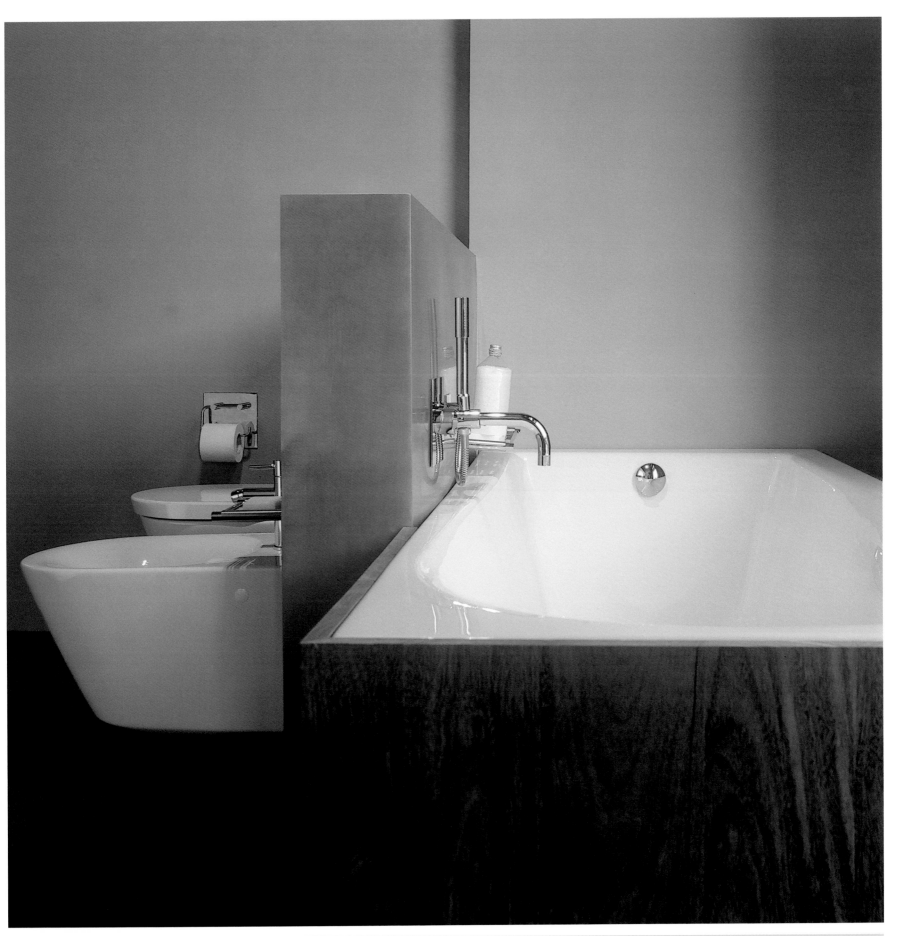

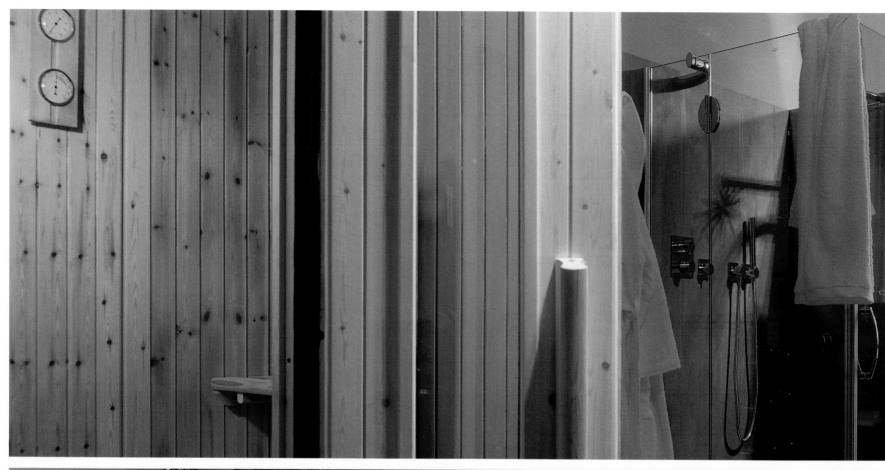

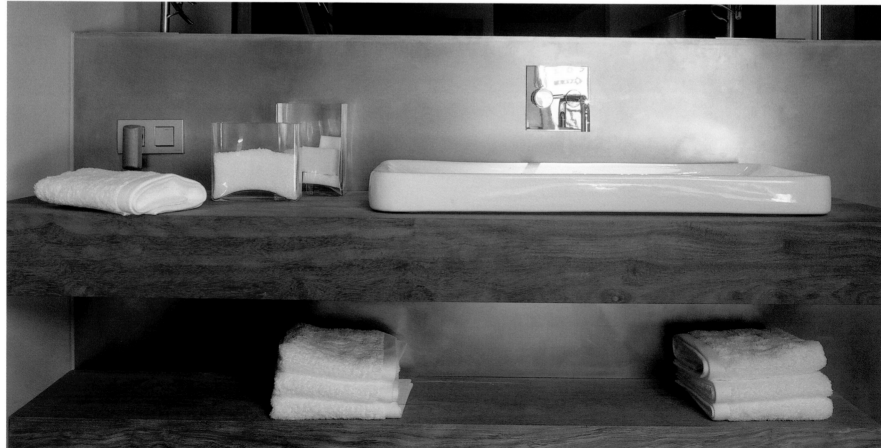

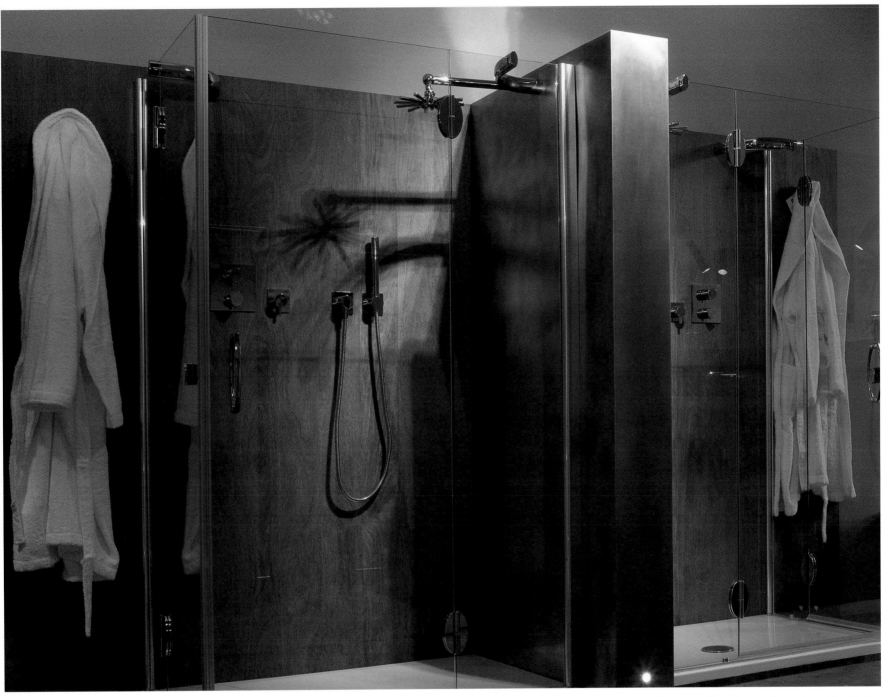

The naturally waterproof wood used inside the showers is resistant to damage.

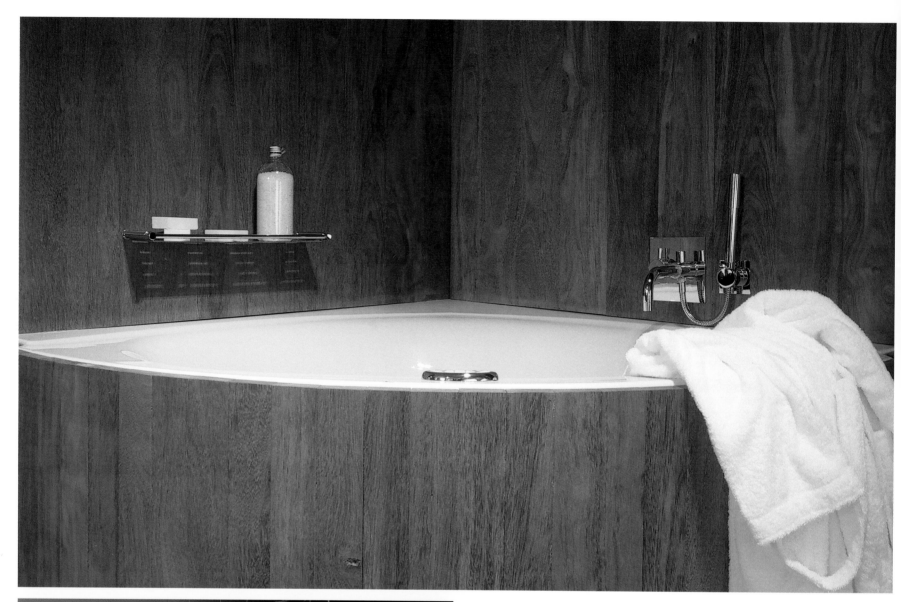

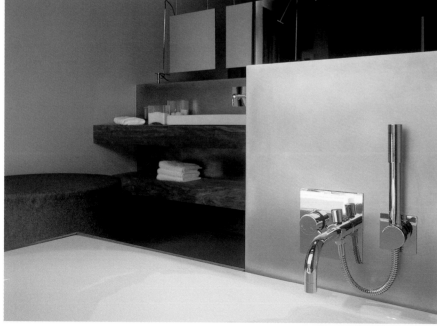

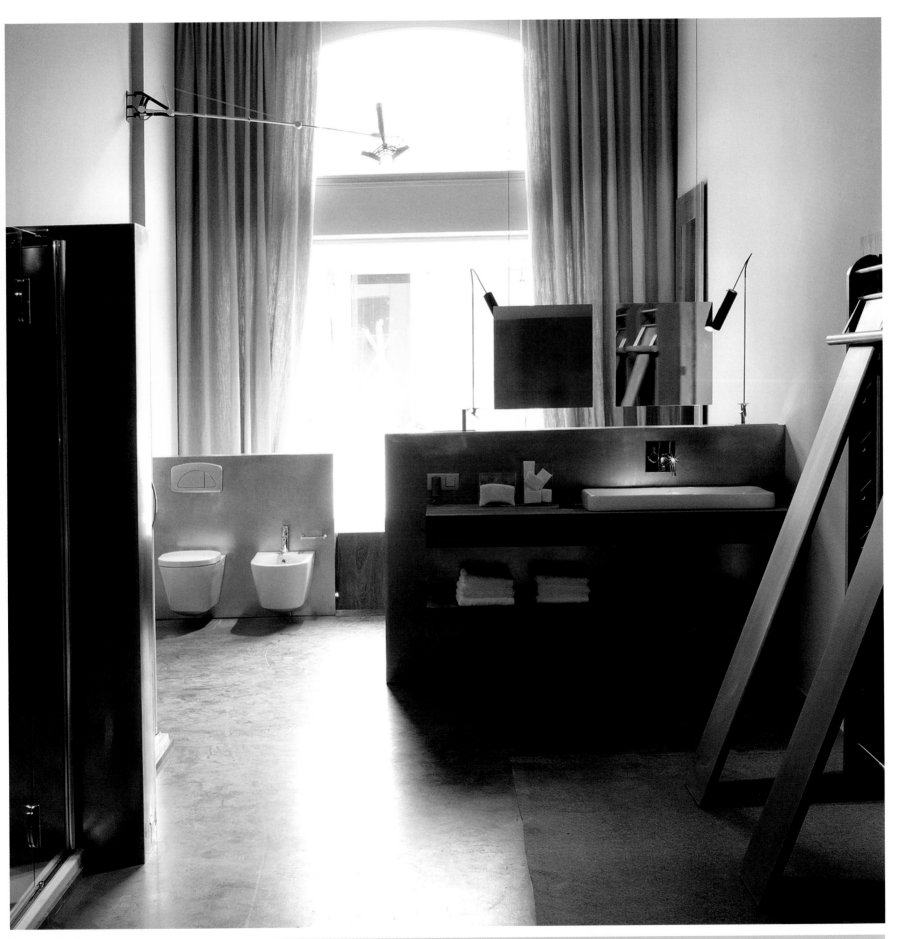

A House
in Bologna

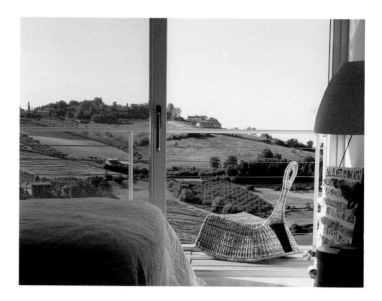

This residence, the home of a famous Italian actor, is nestled onto a hill and enjoys dramatic views of the city of Bologna. Consisting of three levels, it benefits from a spacious bathroom that contains a large hydromassage bath. Its straight lines and the striking amount of natural light that enters the dwelling evoke the baths of ancient Rome. The color white abounds in this light-filled and minimalist space, and the only hints of color come in the form of small green mats and a painting hanging next to the sink. The arrangement of the different elements and the purity and simplicity of the lines create an atmosphere of calm and serenity. There are no superfluous elements to distract one's attention from the most important elements in this room: water and light.

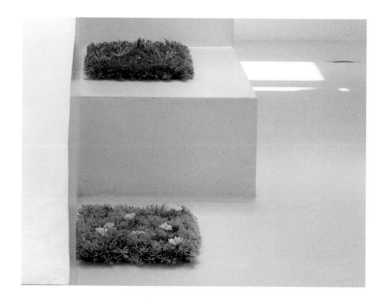

Architect: **Studio Salizzoni**
Location: **Bologna, Italy**
Photos © **Giorgio Possenti/Vega MG**

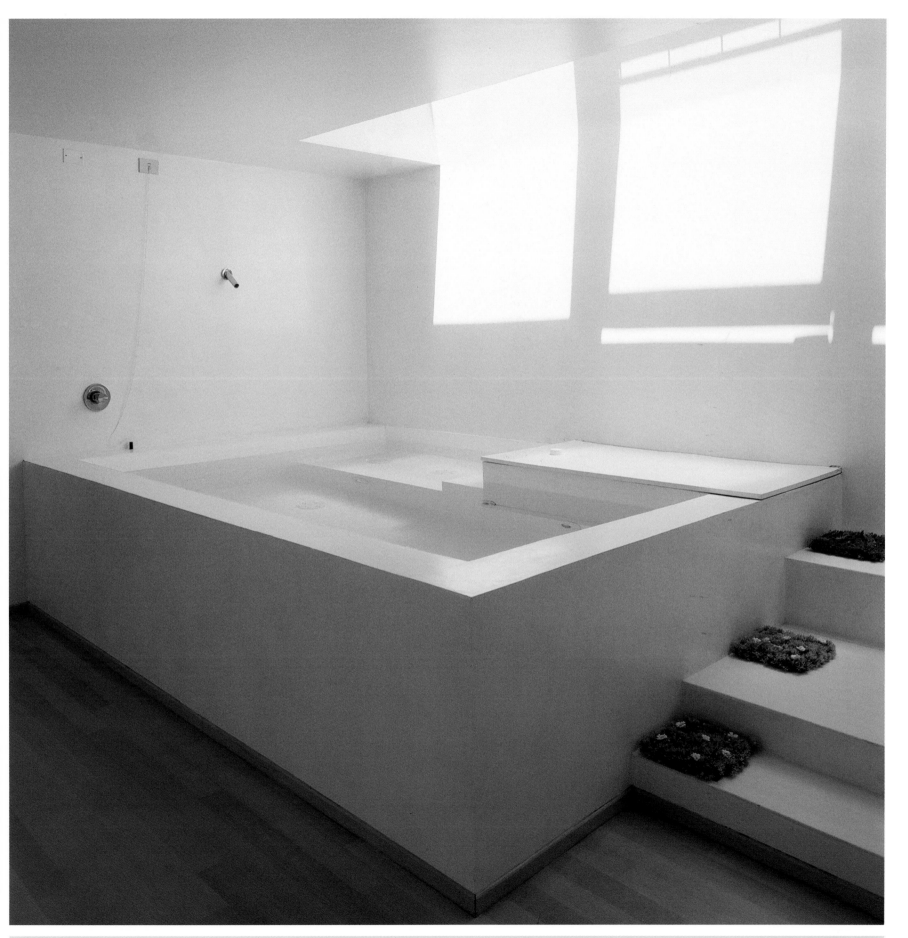

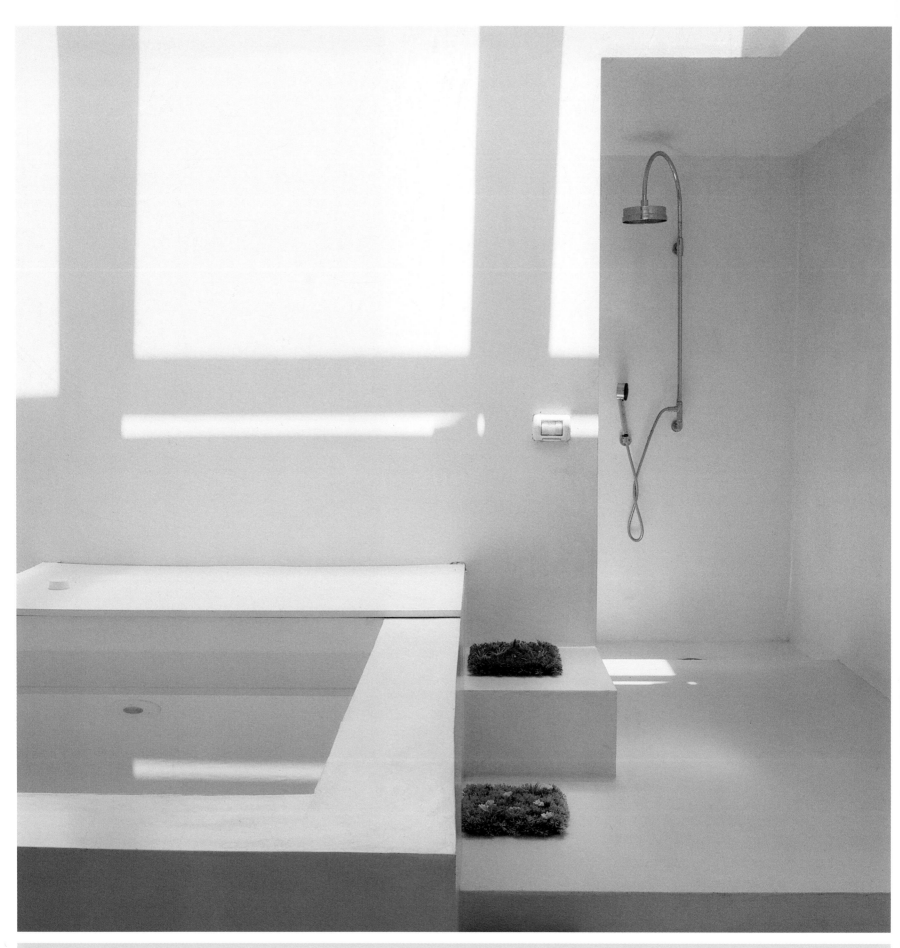

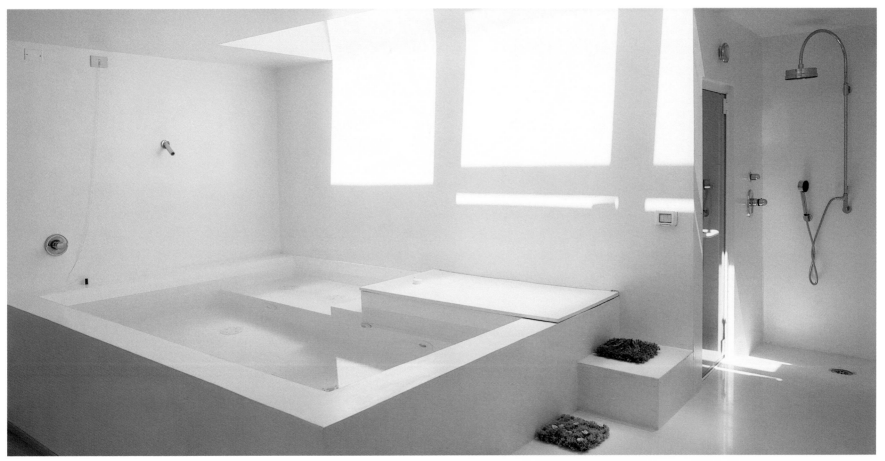

The color white and the natural light that fill this room hark back to the times in which Roman patricians basked in ancient baths.

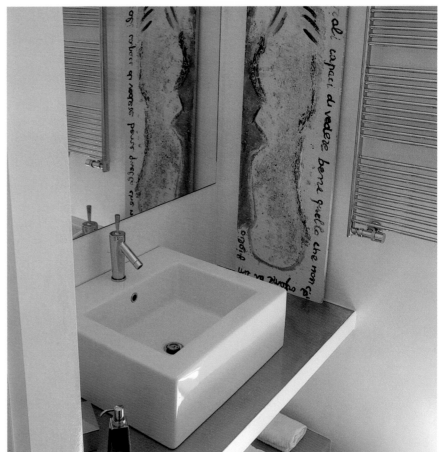

Samadhi Bad Spa

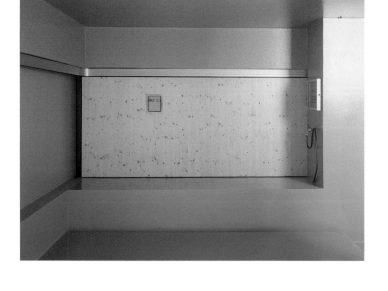

Flotation therapy offers a number of beneficial effects: among other benefits, it relaxes the body, stimulates creativity, enhances one's sleep, and eases muscular pain. Samadhi is a facility equipped with the latest in technology to engage in this therapy, which contributes to one's mental, emotional, and physical well-being. It consists of a multipurpose room that houses the preparatory lounge, the area to relax after bathing, and the flotation tanks themselves, which are differentiated spatially through a scaling back of levels. The flotation is carried out in water that has a very high salt content and at a temperature equivalent to that of the body. The equipment has an automatic system for closing the tank when it is in use, which completely isolates patients from any and all outside stimuli.

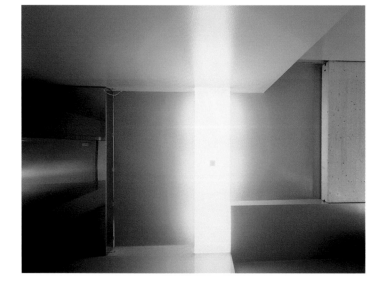

Architect: **Anna Popelka and Georg Poduschka/ PPAG Architekten**
Location: **Graz, Austria**
Photos © **Margherita Spiluttini and Christine Bärnthaler**

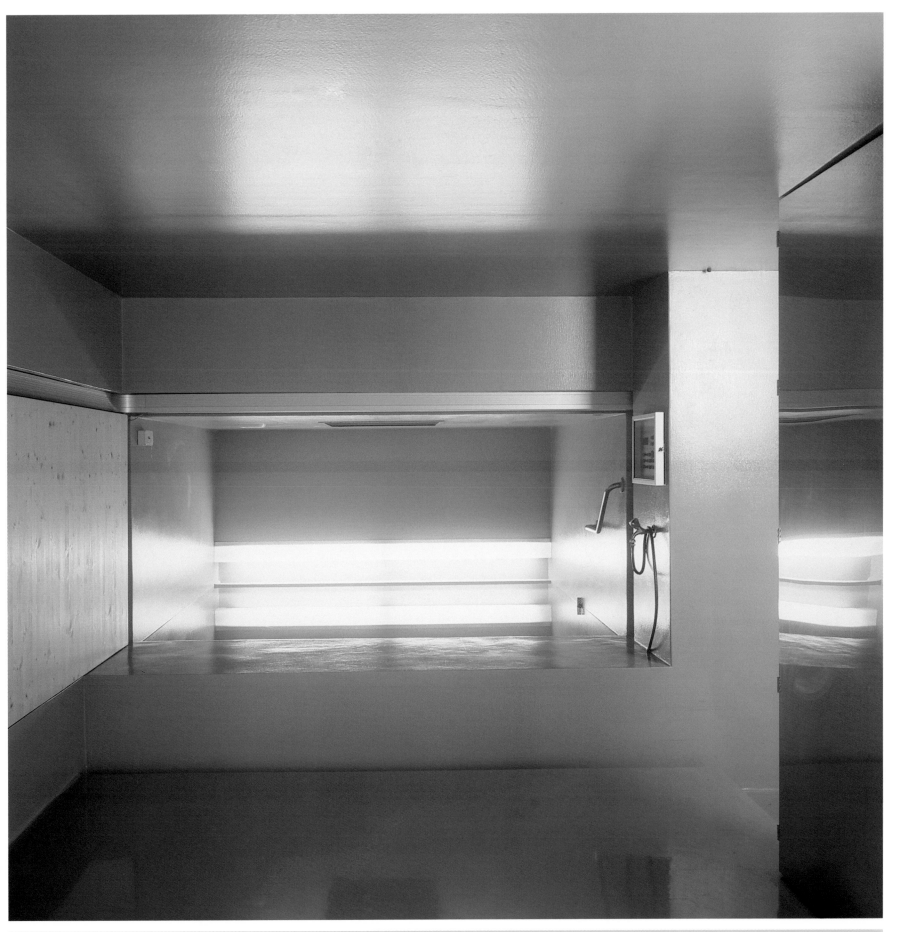

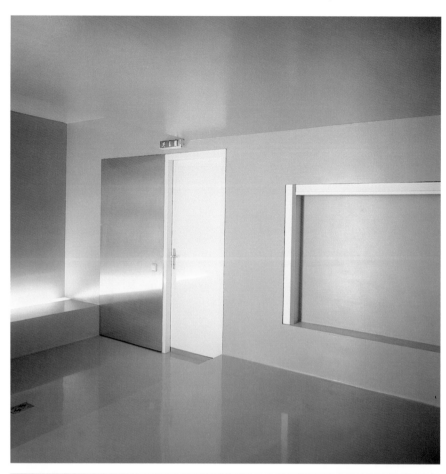

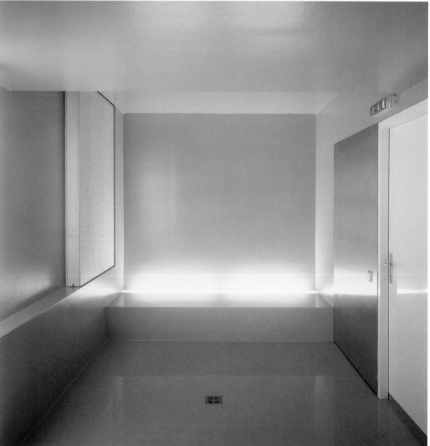

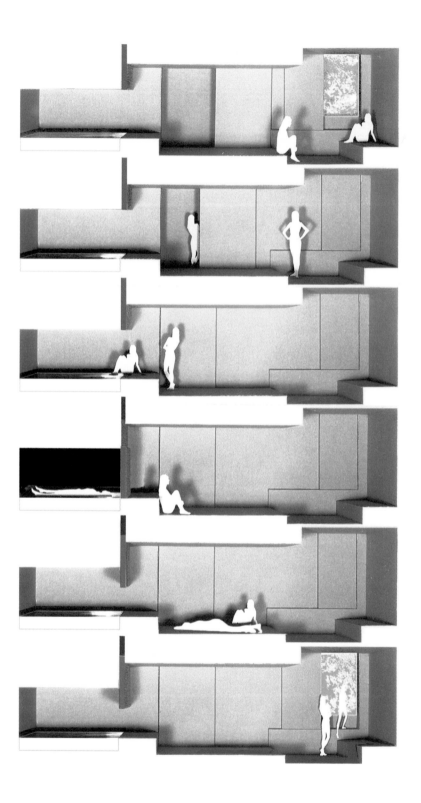

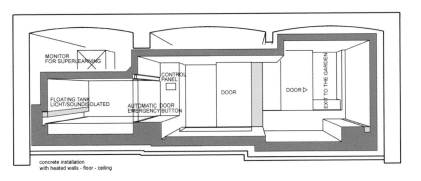

MONITOR
FOR SUPERLEARNING

CONTROL
PANEL

FLOATING TANK
LICHT/SOUNDISOLATED

AUTOMATIC DOOR
EMERGENCY BUTTON

DOOR

DOOR ▷

EXIT TO THE GARDEN

concrete installation
with heated walls - floor - ceiling

Section

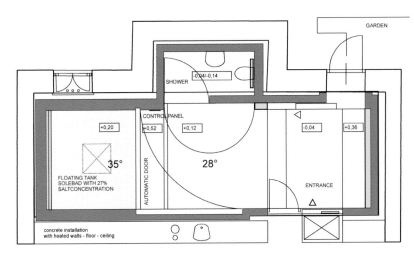

GARDEN

SHOWER

-0,04/-0,14

CONTROL PANEL

+0,20

+0,52

+0,12

-0,04

+0,36

35°

28°

FLOATING TANK
SOLEBAD WITH 27%
SALTCONCENTRATION

AUTOMATIC DOOR

ENTRANCE

concrete installation
with heated walls - floor - ceiling

Basement

The wooden door allows one to close off the tank,
which grants the user a tremendous degree of
tranquility to enjoy the moment of floating.

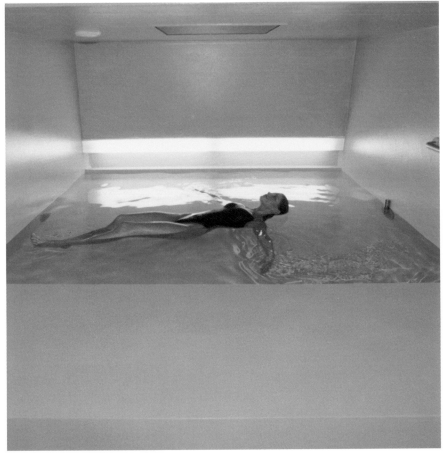

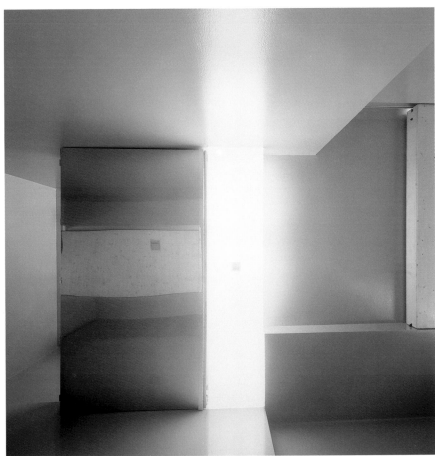

A Pool
in Carefree

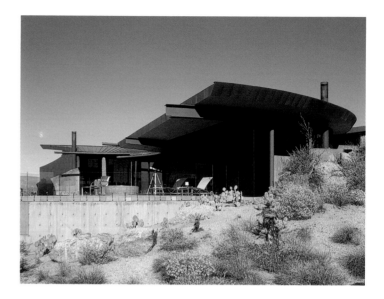

The cactus gives away the location of this circular spa, located in Arizona, which is home to a very hot climate. The pool and hydro-massage bath represent an excellent solution for both combating the heat and enjoying the outdoors. The house, nestled into a sloping site, consists of a terraced design to respect the topography. Cement, which is the predominant material throughout, is also present in the hydromassage bath, lending the spa and the rest of the architecture a sober and elegant air. The pool allows one to go for a refreshing dip, and from the bath, situated on a higher level, one can contemplate the landscape as well as breathtaking sunsets. The hammocks and cactuses are practically the only elements decorating this unique, curving terrace of ample proportions. The space it creates is a perfect place for relaxing and escaping from the stresses and pressure of everyday routines.

Architect: **Jones Studio**
Location: **Carefree, Arizona, United States**
Photos © **Pere Planells**

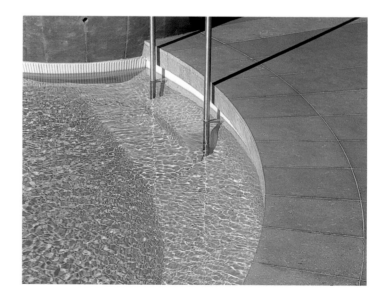

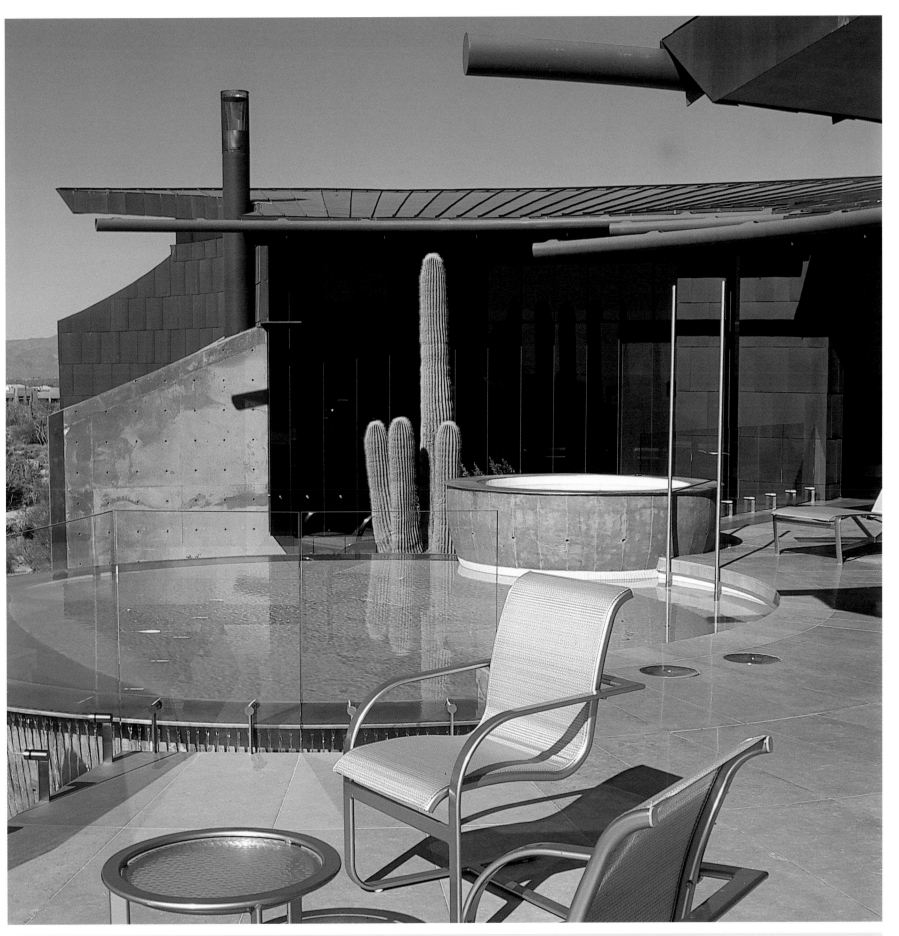

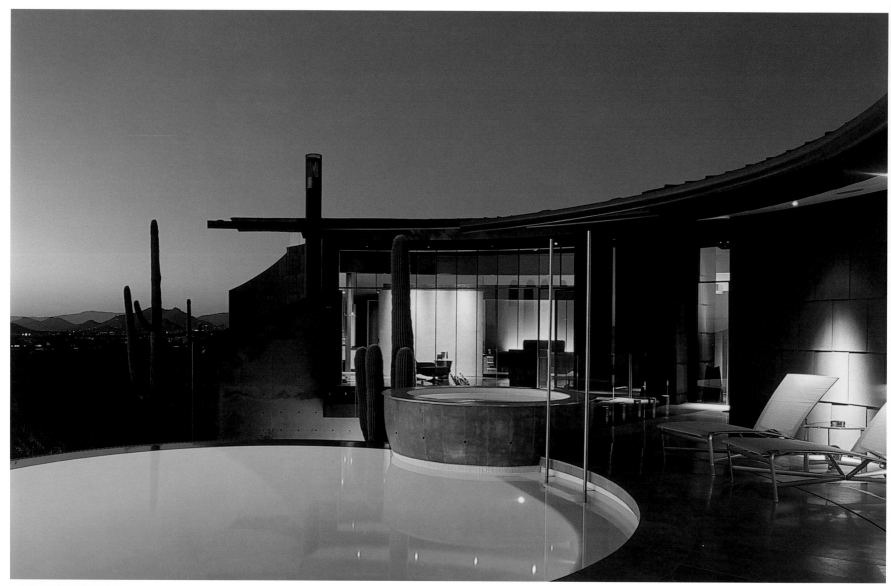

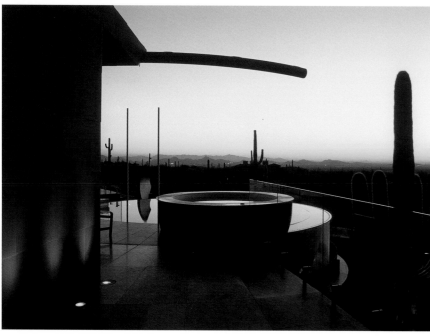

The bath is located on a different level than the pool, which allows one to indulge in a private hydromassage while taking in spectacular views.

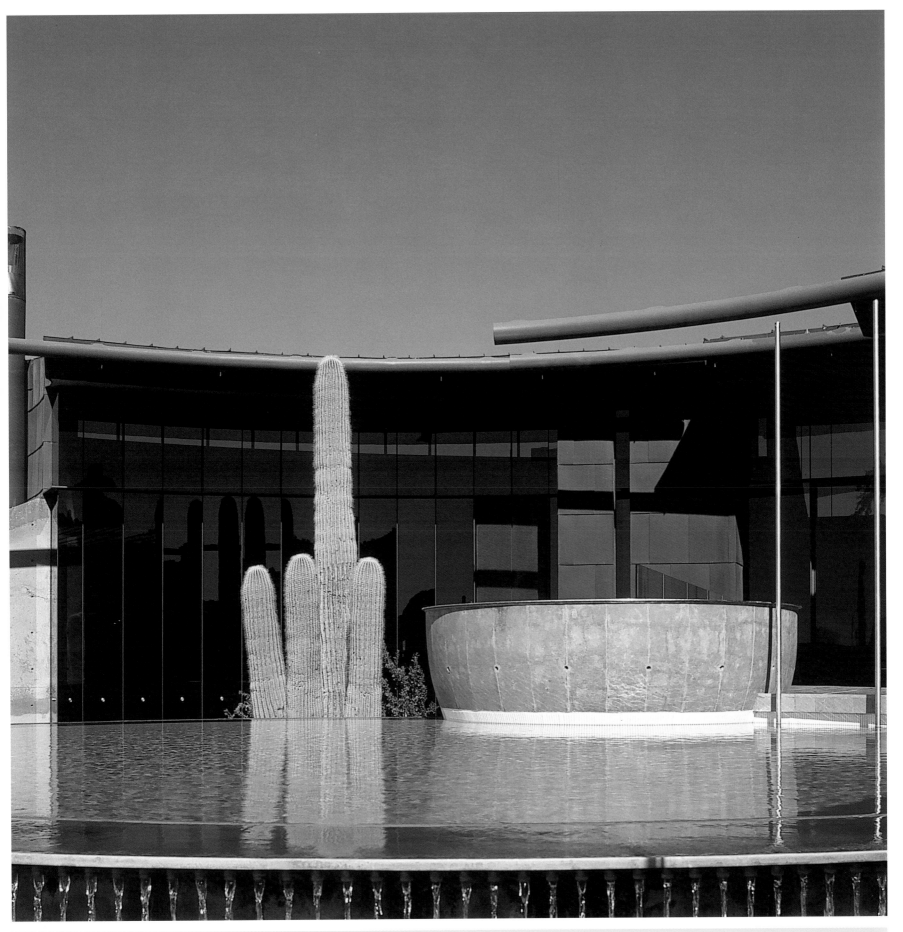

Machiya House

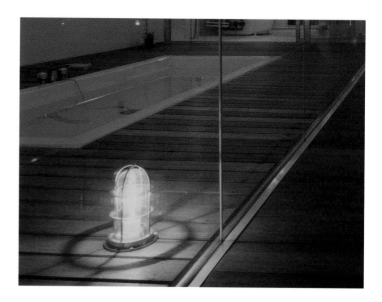

The architecture of this house plays with the concepts of interior and exterior: the courtyards around the house are delimited by sliding glass walls that purposefully blur its limits. This visual continuity, together with the extraordinary amount of light entering the house, enhances the sensation of spaciousness. A bath is located in one of these courtyards and is built into the floor. This bath, in turn, can be accessed from the main bathroom, which contains another bath with a hydromassage, a multifunction toilet, a shower, and a sink. Japanese tradition stresses the importance of the ritual of bathing, as it is viewed as a necessary condition to achieving well-being. The ambience created by this *ofuro* is especially warm and filled with light: the wooden floors ensure comfort, while white canvas awnings can be adjusted to cover the spa and create a more intimate and quiet ambience.

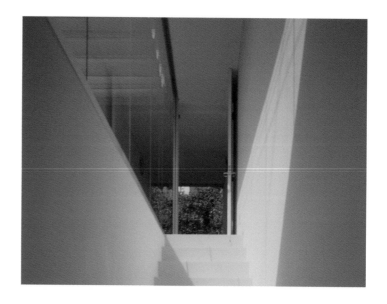

Architect: **Takaharu + Yiu Tezuka/Tezuka Architects, Masahiro Ikeda/mias**
Location: **Tokyo, Japan**
Lighting Design: **Masahide Kakudate/Masahide Kakudate Lighting Architect & Associates**
Lighting Photos © **Katsuhisa Kida Photography**

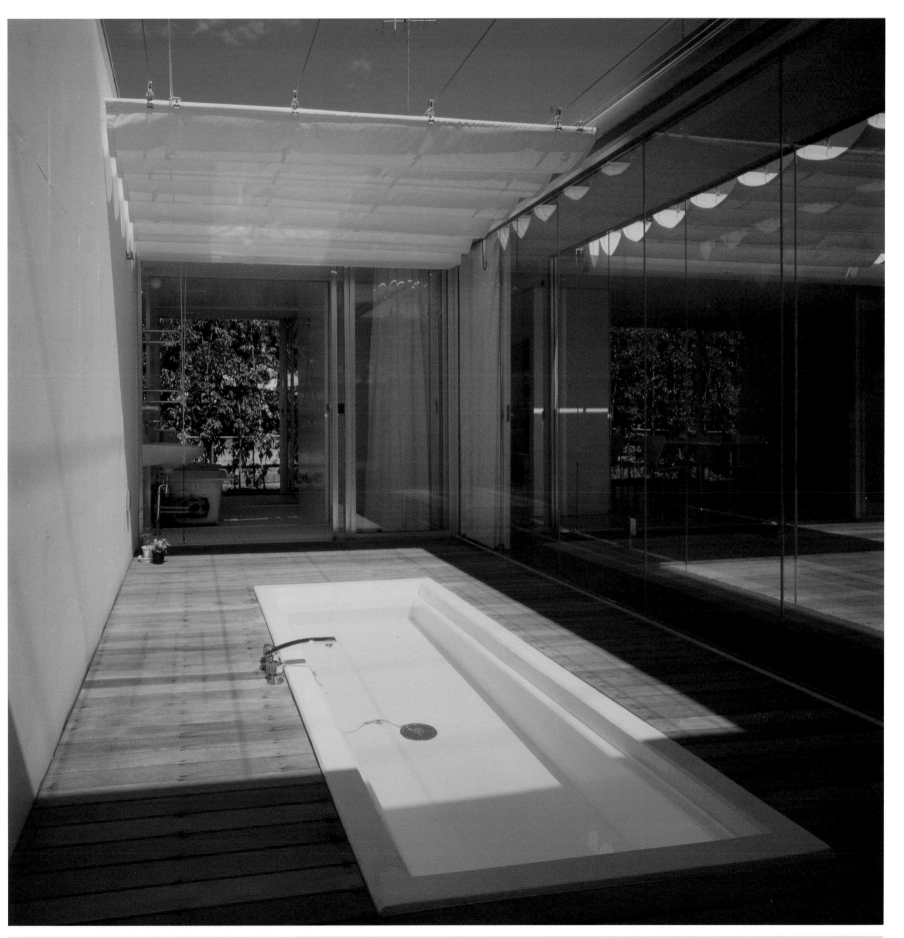

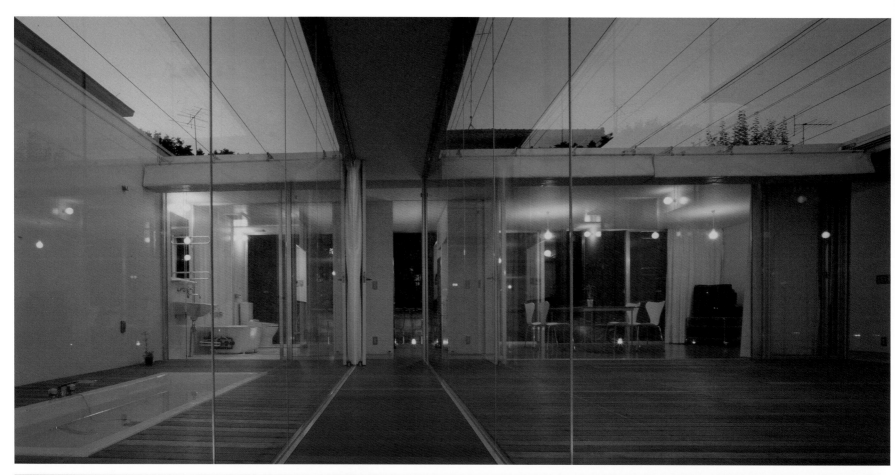

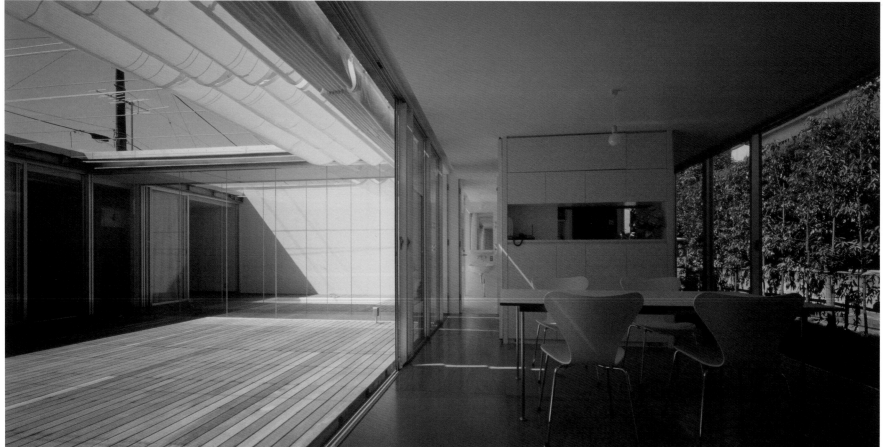

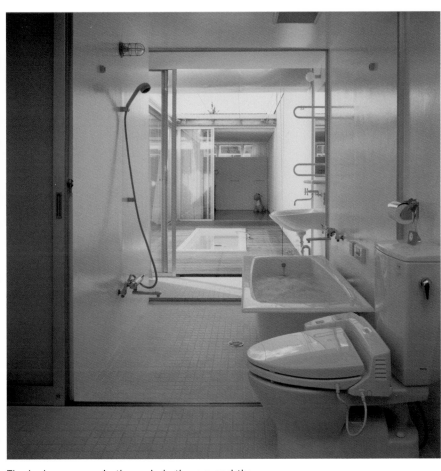

The hydromassage in the main bathroom and the outdoor bath are the main elements in this spa, which rethinks the Japanese concept of the *ofuro*.

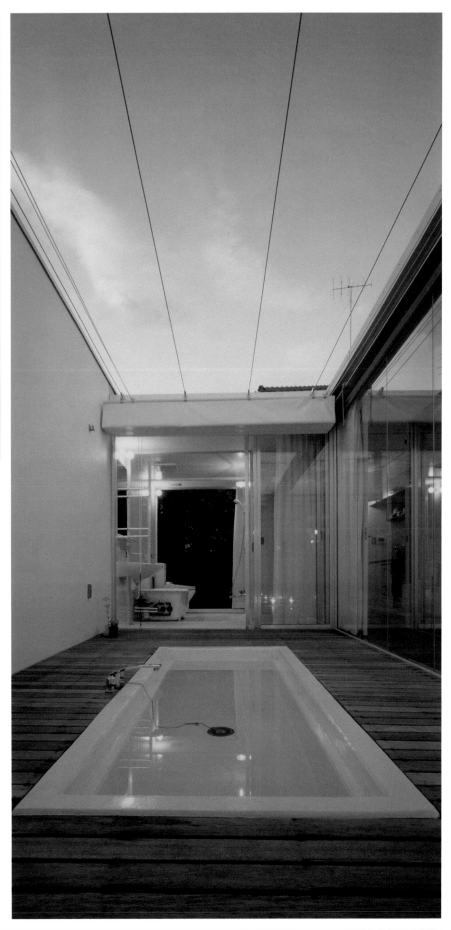

A Gymnasium in Milan

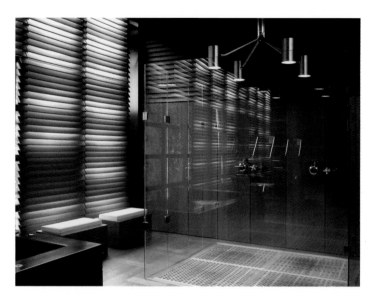

This spectacular facility, designed by Studiomonti, is a gymnasium that is clearly divided into two areas: the first is for machines and weights, while the second is designed for relaxation and contains a glass shower cubicle with room for several people and a large hydromassage bath, designed by the architects themselves. On the wall alongside the bath there is a mural—made up of plasma screens—which can be adjusted to easily change the aesthetic of the room. In fact, from the bath, one can effortlessly engage in contemplating the changing images, listening to music, or watching television. The entire perimeter of the interior is lined in wooden slats, which—despite the modern design—provide for a warm and welcoming environment. The lighting was meticulously designed throughout to strengthen the character of the space. In the shower, for example, a lighting system was installed in the showerheads themselves, so that the cascading water is always illuminated. This constantly changing atmosphere enhances both exercise and relaxation.

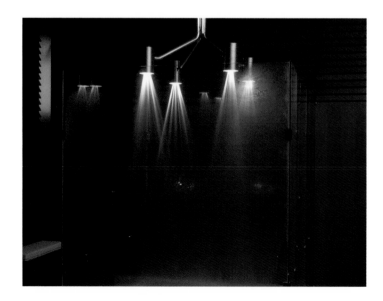

Architect: **Studiomonti**
Location: **Milan, Italy**
Photos © **Alessandro Ciampi**

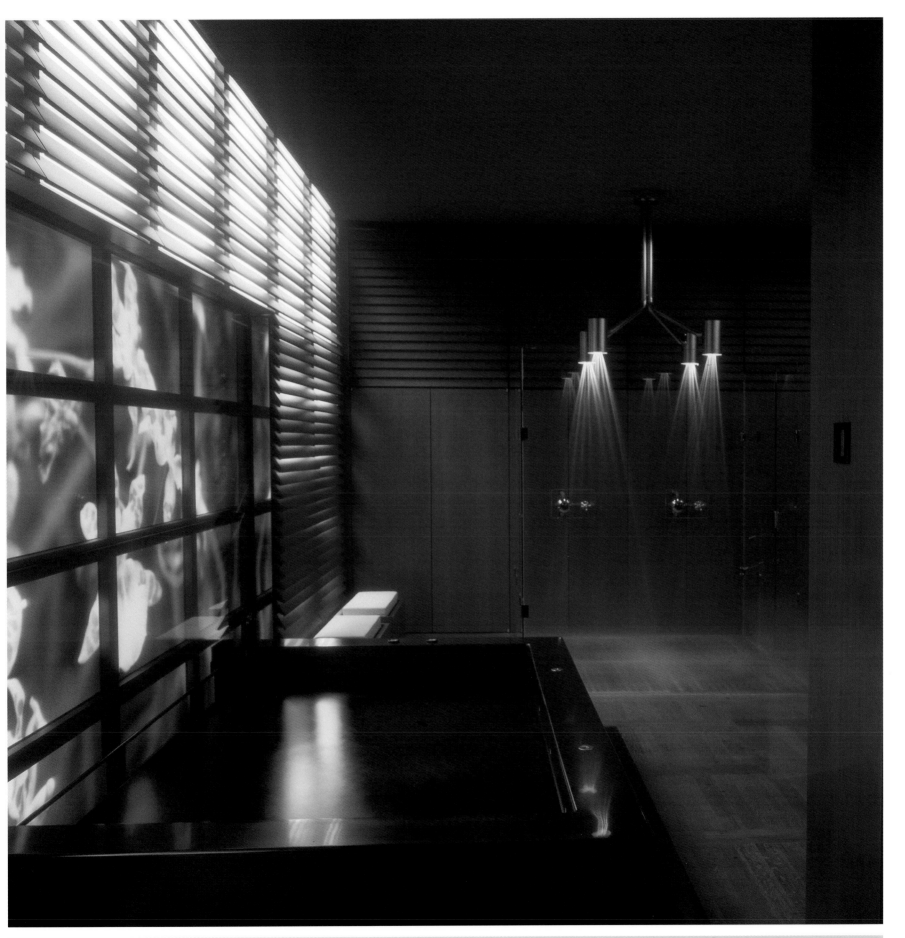

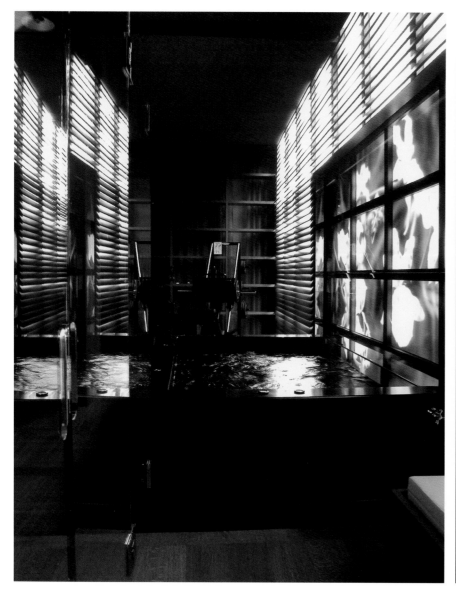

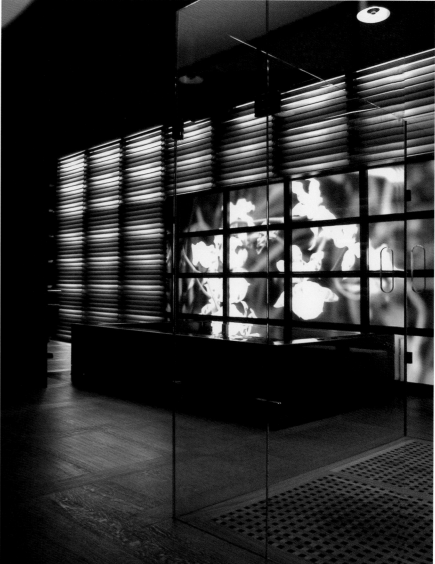

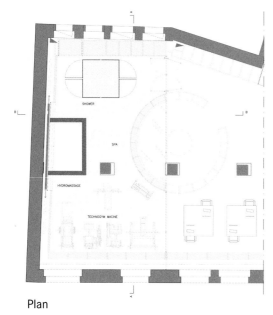

Plan

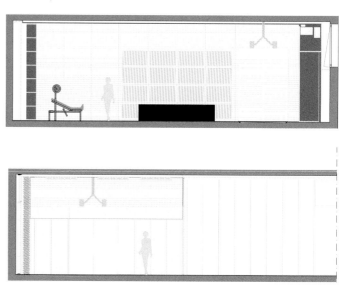

Sections

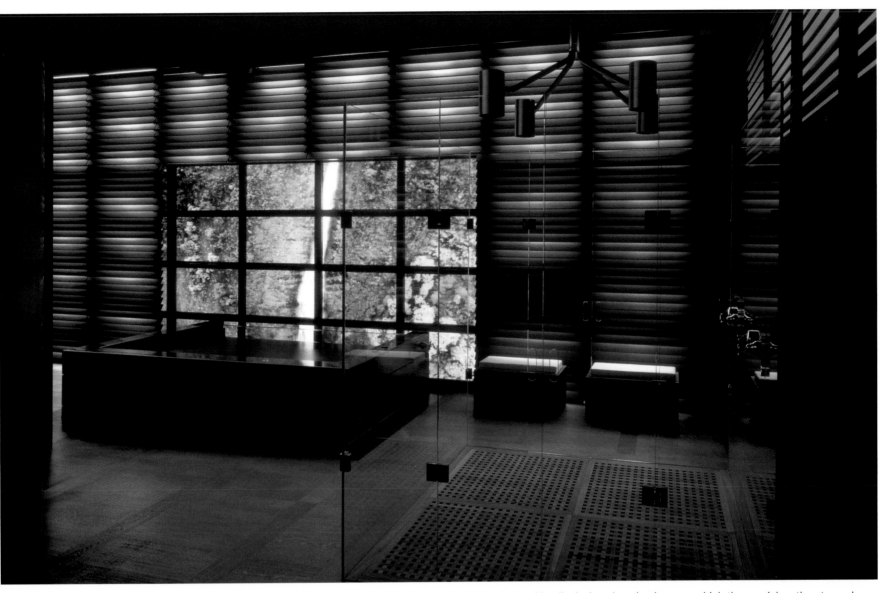

The plasma-screen mural allows the ambience of the room to be changed by displaying changing images, which thus enriches the atmosphere.

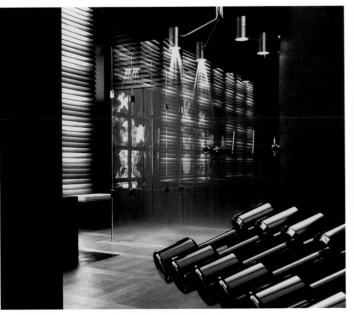

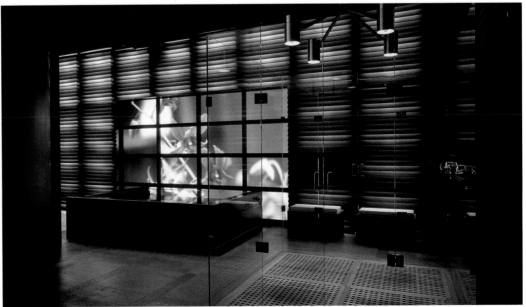

A Spa on Central Park

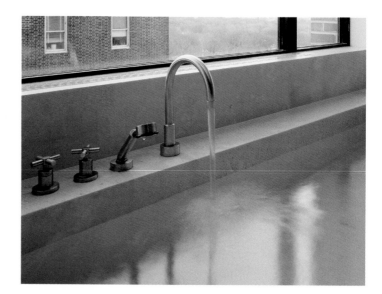

The renovation of this 7,500-square-foot apartment located in Manhattan sheds light on its owner's philosophy of life: it includes a generously sized bathroom, which is flooded with natural light, and enjoys breathtaking views out over Central Park. It was designed to permit meditation as well as to allow one to enjoy a relaxing bath. The entire house is thus impregnated with this spirit: the floor in the master bedroom resembles tatami mats, and a special floor was installed in another room to allow one to practice yoga. Shades of ivory and teak lend a serene, minimalist air, and the small Asian-inspired details define a décor that eschews excess. The area of the spa is connected to the master bedroom and to one of the terraces that extend around the apartment. This generates the privacy and independence that one needs to be able to rest, reflect, and recover one's internal equilibrium and peace.

Architect: **Bonetti Kozerski Studio**
Location: **New York City, United States**
Photos © **Matteo Piazza**

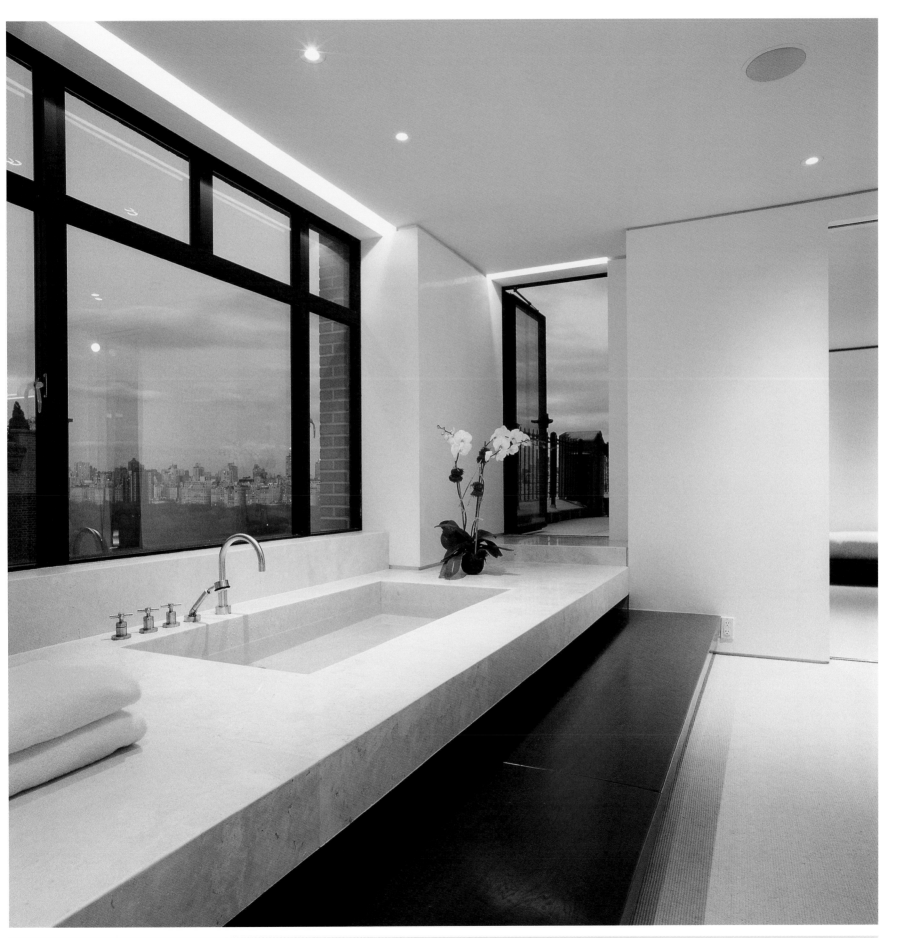

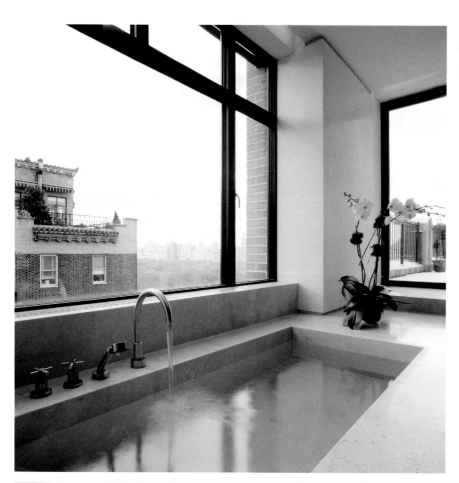

From the area of the bath, situated next to a large window, one can access the terrace, which extends nearly all the way around the apartment.

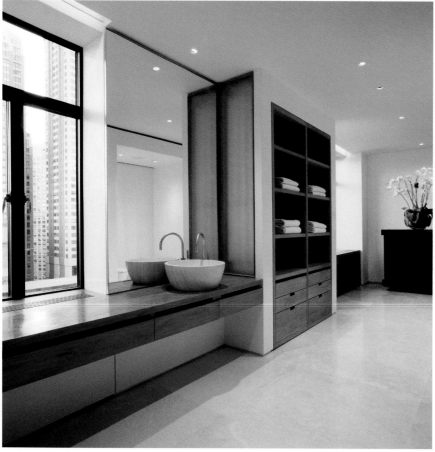

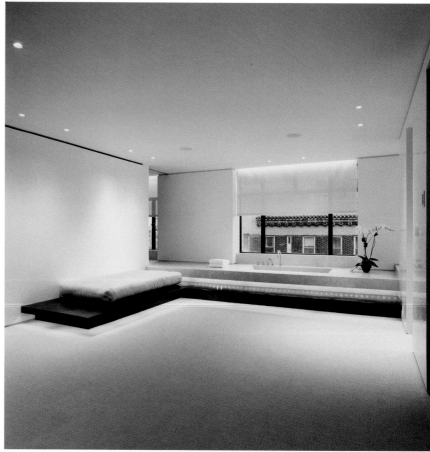

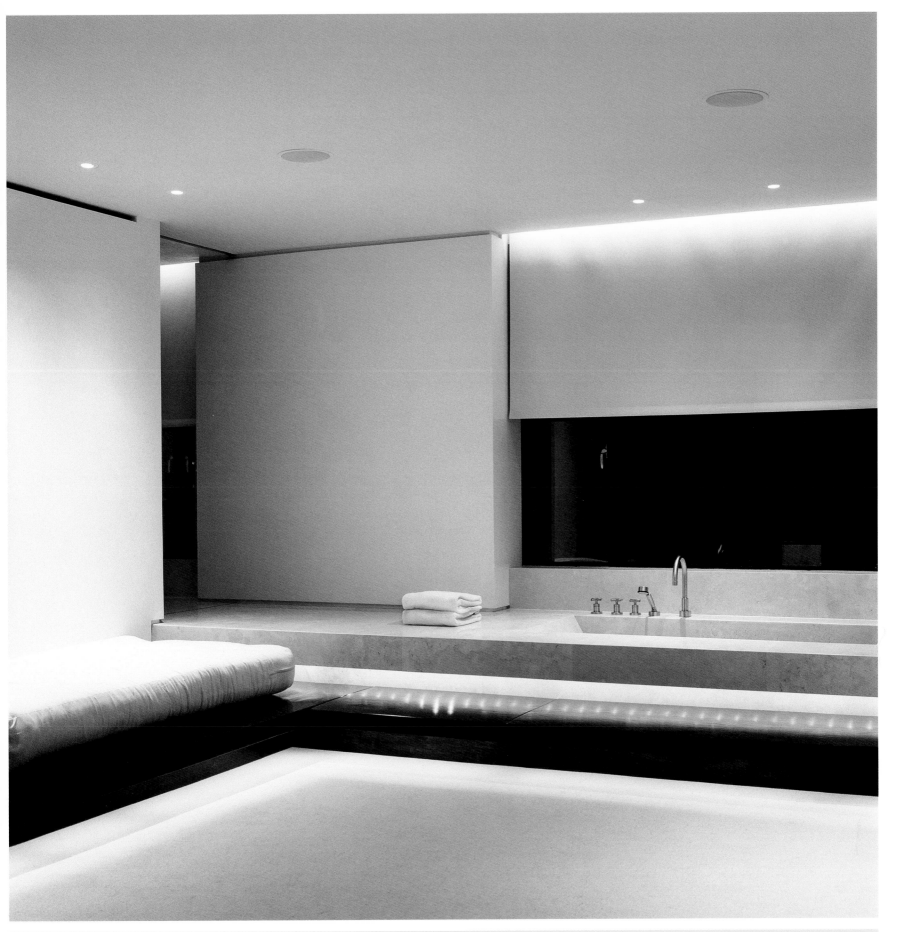

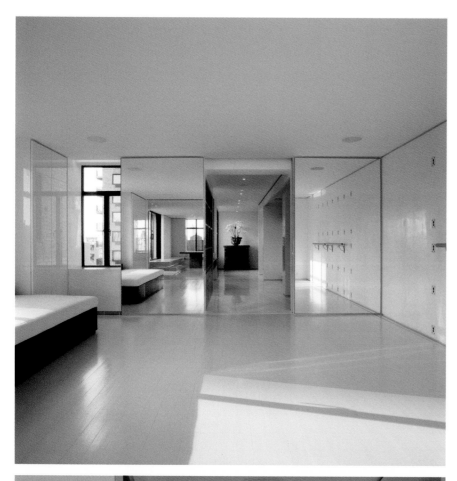

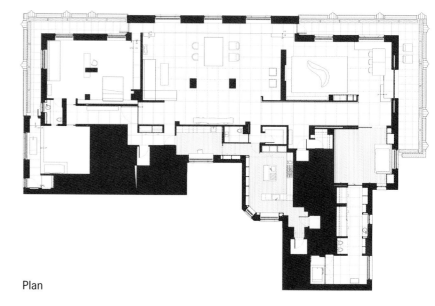

Plan

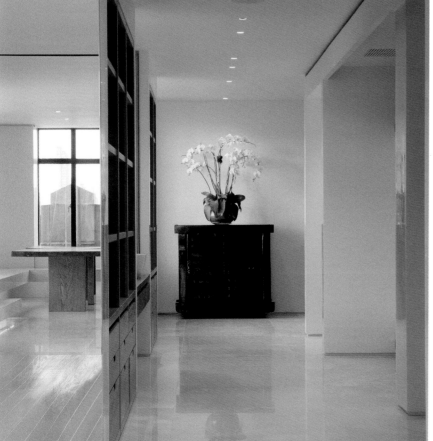

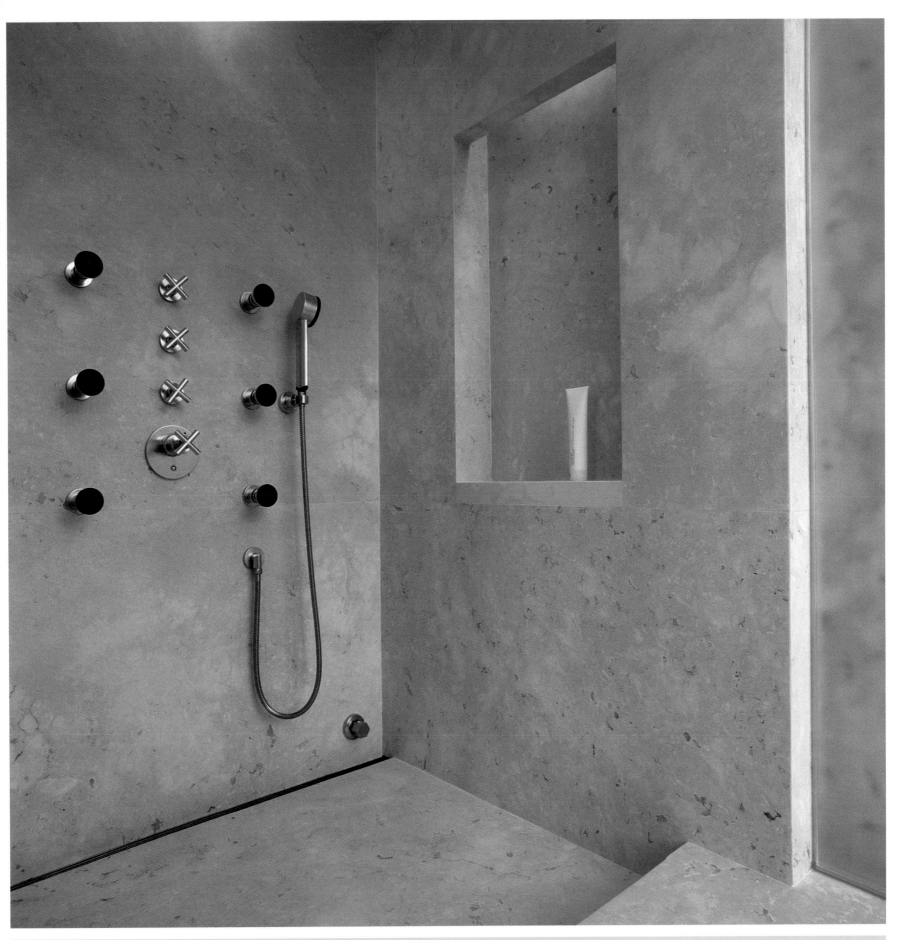

An Apartment on Grosvenor Street

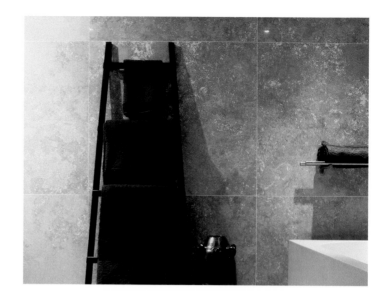

This carefully designed apartment in London benefits from the inclusion of an equally elegant spa, whose various zones—powder room, shower, and toilet—conserve their inhabitants' privacy behind wood and glass doors, yet do not interrupt the spatial unity of the home. The shower—replete with hydromassage—and the large, free-standing bath are the two pieces that duel for one's attention in the room; one is struck with the dilemma of whether to take a revitalizing shower or a relaxing bath. The dark tones of the wood furniture stand in contrast to the white walls and bathroom fixtures, and this contrast further serves to highlight the quality of all the materials used. Current trends, which place a greater emphasis on the bath inside the home, are evident in this oasis of cleanliness and relaxation.

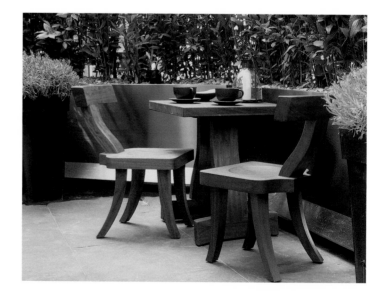

Decorators: **Candy & Candy**
Location: **London, United Kingdom**
Photos © **Andreas von Einsiedel**

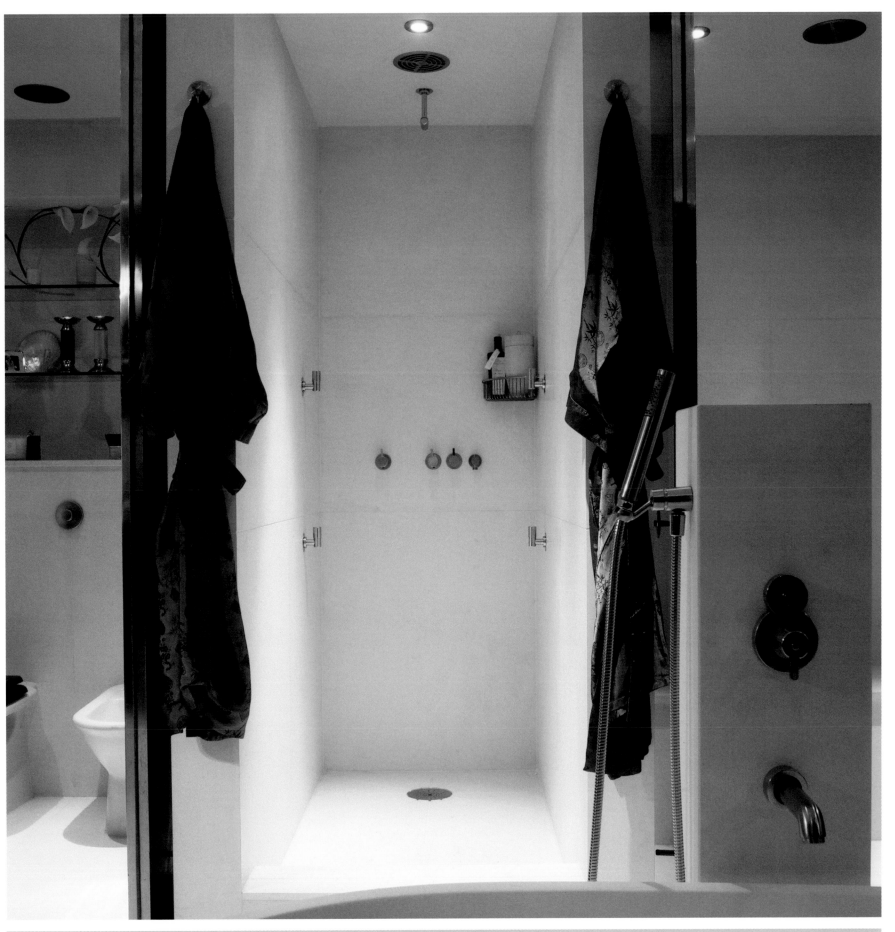

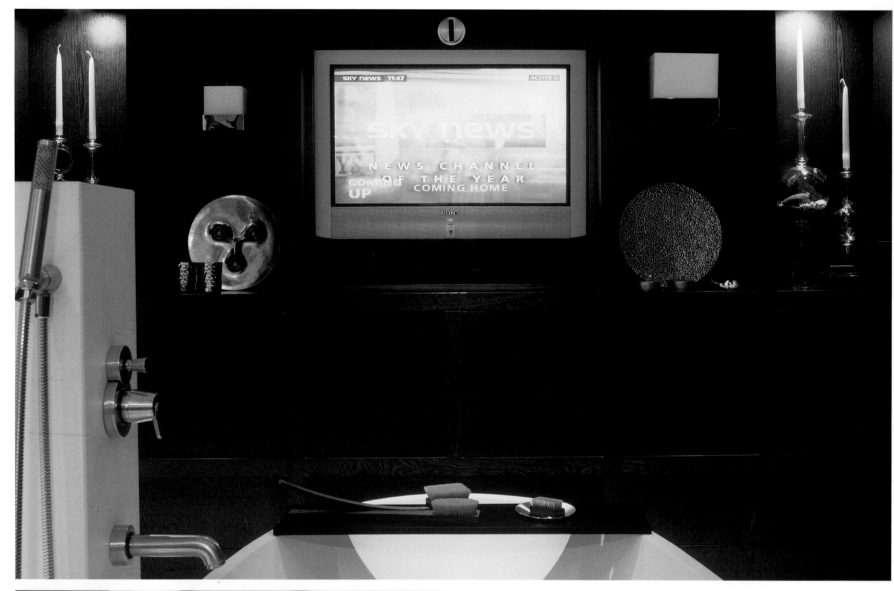

The built-in plasma-screen television allows one the opportunity to enjoy a film while taking a relaxing bath.

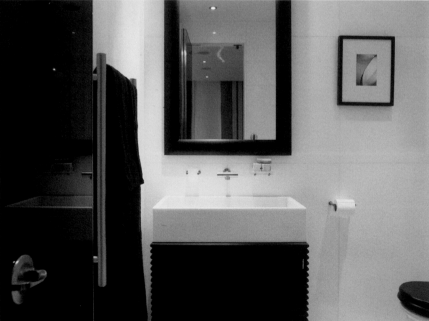

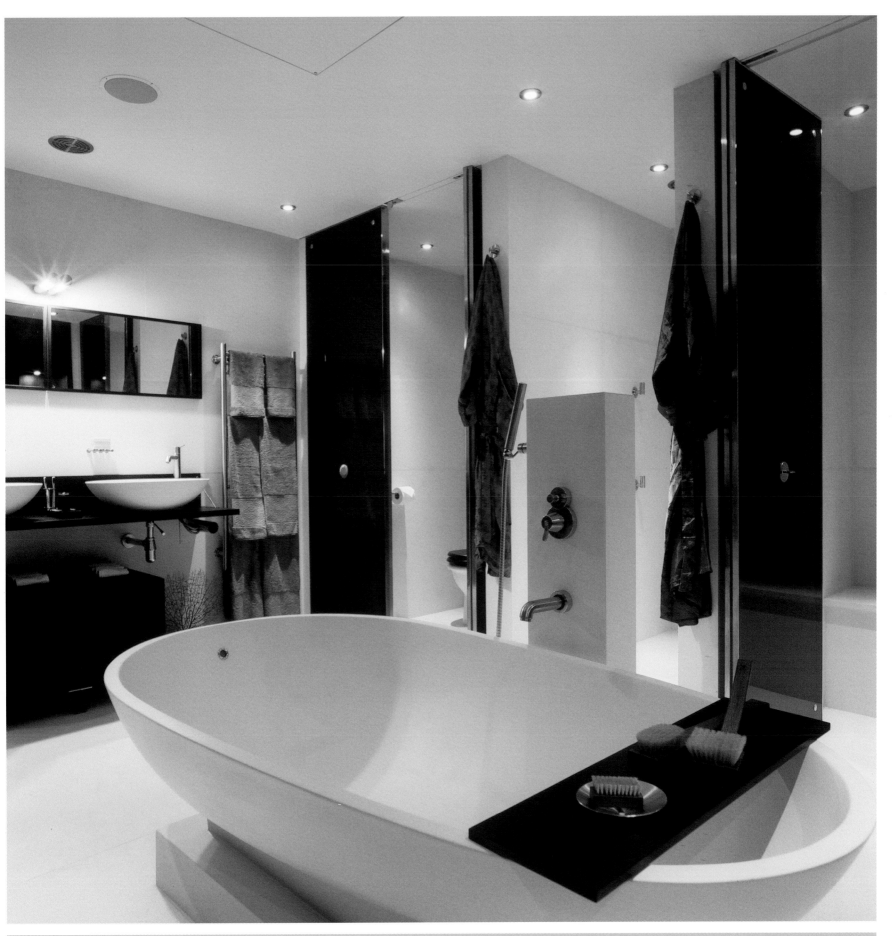

Casa Lloreda

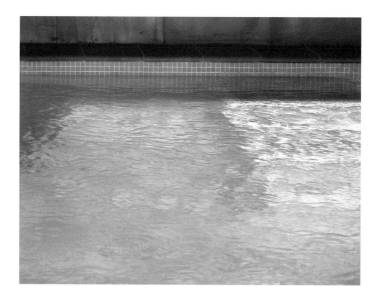

This spa was built with two clear objectives in mind: first, to provide a place for the owners to relax and get away to, and second, to design a place that could be enjoyed year round. To this end, a pavilion was built that would open onto an outdoor garden and porch, which houses a pool and a hexagonal hydromassage bath. In addition to representing an ideal environment in which the owners could decompress from the stress of their jobs, this getaway allows the couple to share moments of everyday conversation. A large window gives way to a flood of natural light, which fills the house with light and calm all day long. The materials used throughout the pavilion respect the natural colors of the surrounding landscape and provide it with a feeling of warmth. The small tiles in the pool are very light in color to highlight the transparency of the water. The slate wall brings nature indoors, while the wood details forge a warm atmosphere.

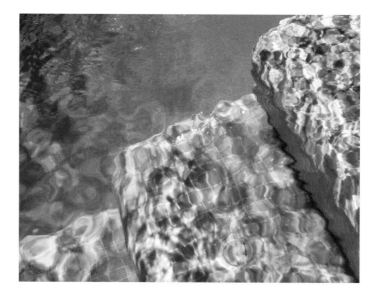

Architect: **Caña y Caña**
Designer: **Elena Surribas**
Location: **Les Franqueses del Vallès, Barcelona, Spain**
Photos © **Thomas Wagner**

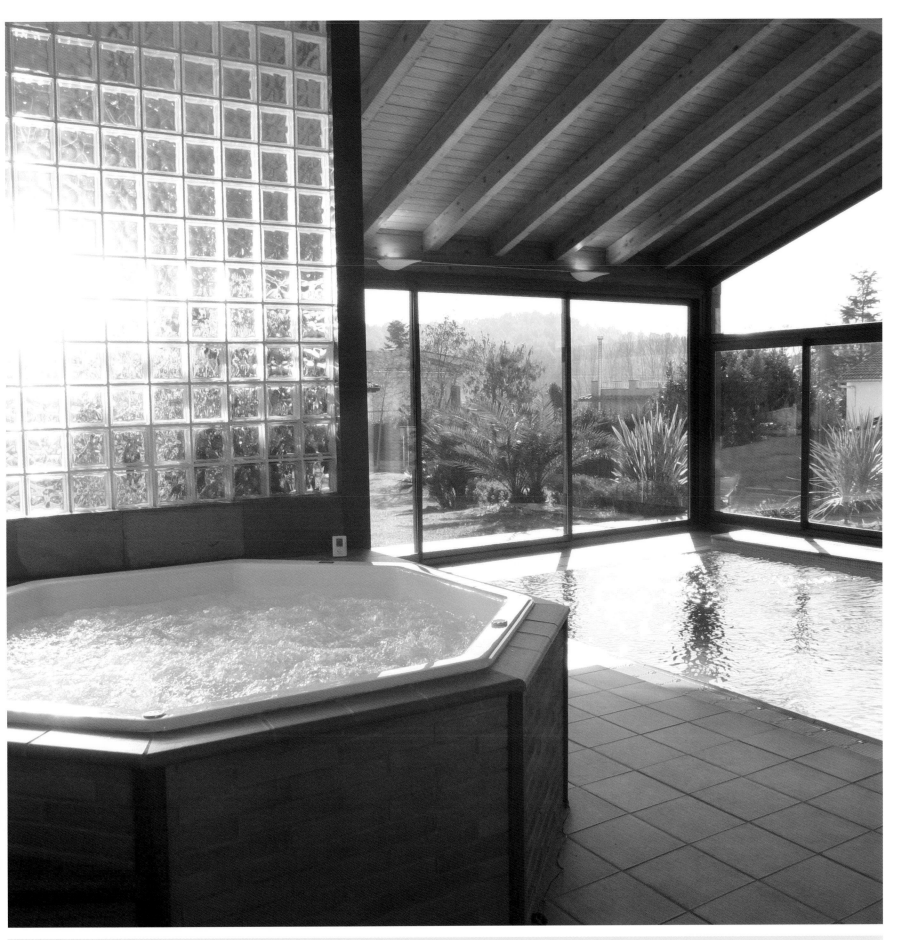

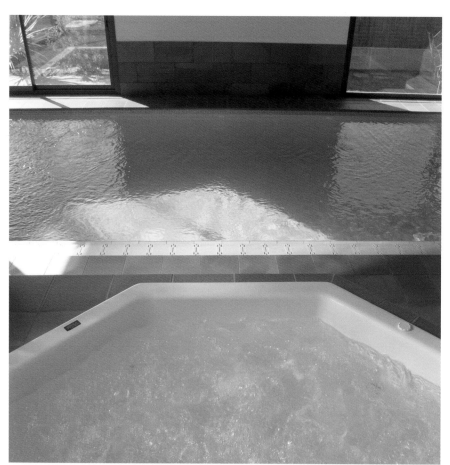

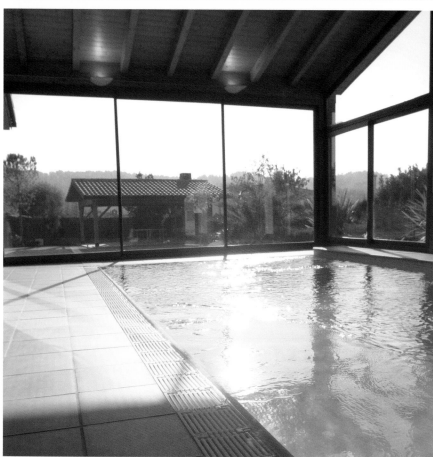

The light tones inside the pool grant the water a greater degree of transparency—it appears to be a crystalline blue.

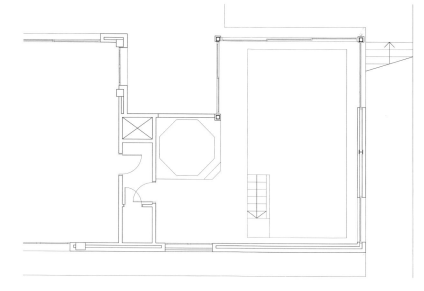

Plan

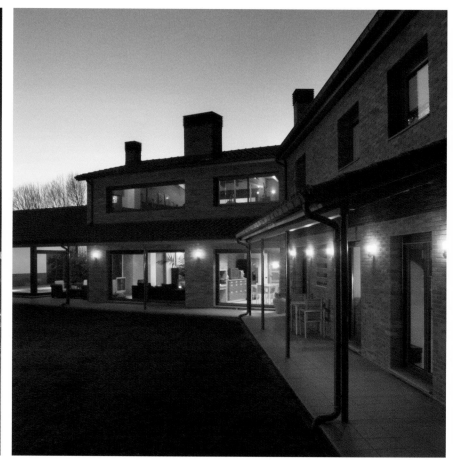

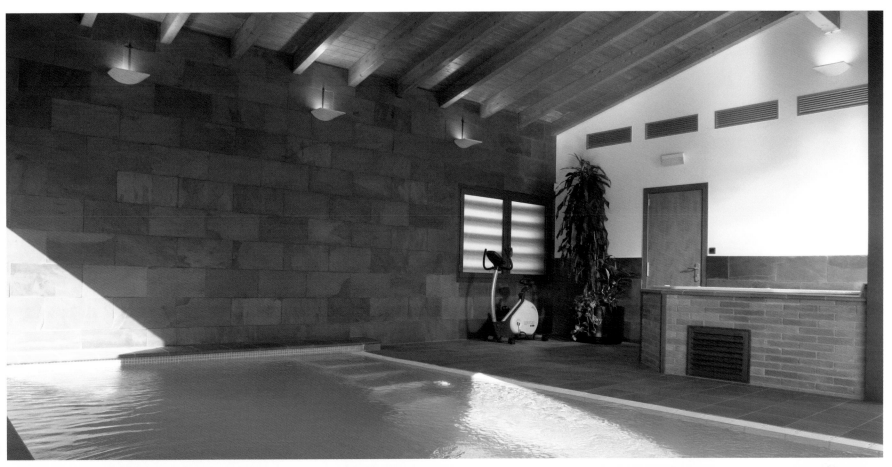

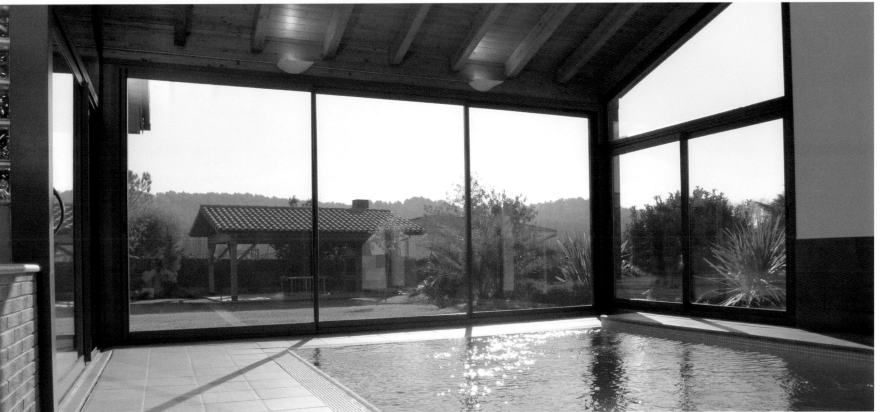

A large window in one of the walls—which fills the spa with even more light—makes this space unique and highlights the simplicity of its lines.

A Spa in
Beverly Hills

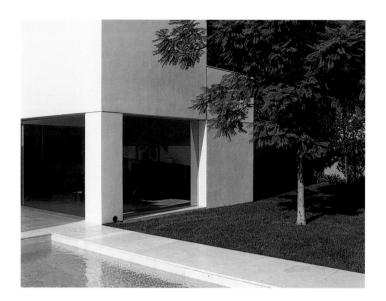

The area that houses this residence's outdoor spa is an elegant and light-filled space. This project, with its contemporary touches and perfect finishes, gives off an air of orderliness and serenity, thanks to the layout of the hydromassage bath and the pool—these represent the main elements on this spacious terrace. The round shape of the bath contrasts with the straight lines of the pool and the architecture of the house. Travertine from Navona was chosen as the main decorative element and was used to frame and unify the water area. The white of the house and the marble grants a feeling of spaciousness and brightness to this terrace, which is furthermore surrounded by a carefully cared-for garden to enhance the feeling of calm. The furnishings that were chosen—two hammocks, a sofa, and a small table—were crafted in natural materials to lend warmth to this immaculate place.

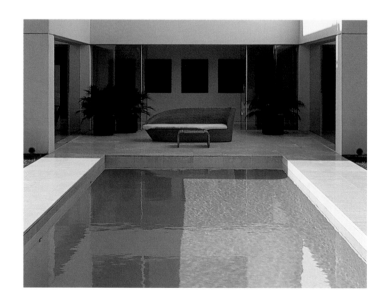

Architect: **Moisés Becker**
Location: **Beverly Hills, California, United States**
Photos © **Pere Planells**

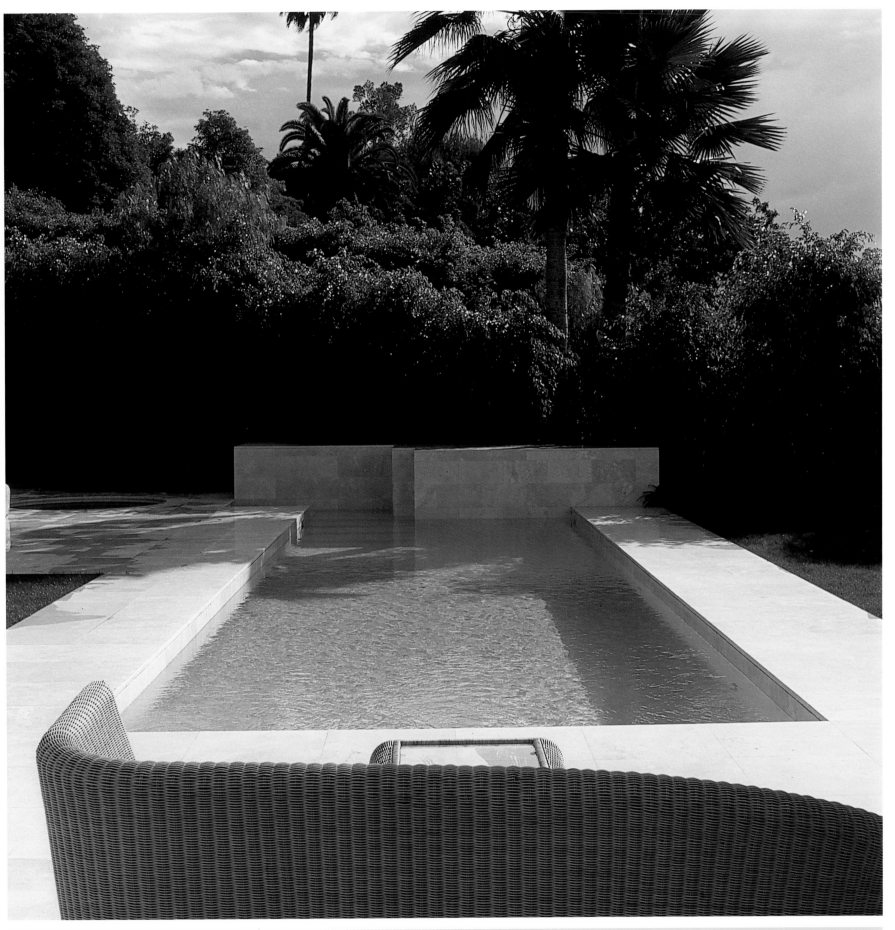

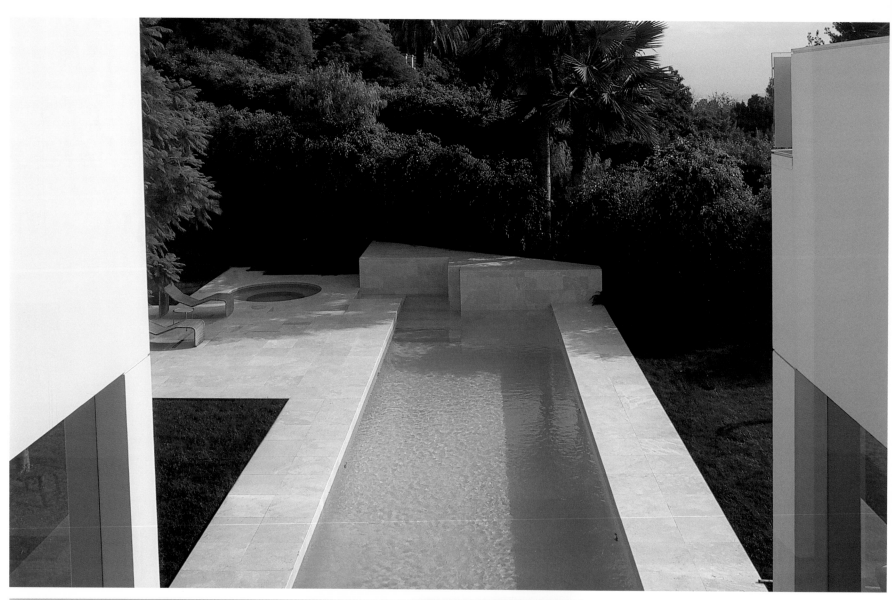

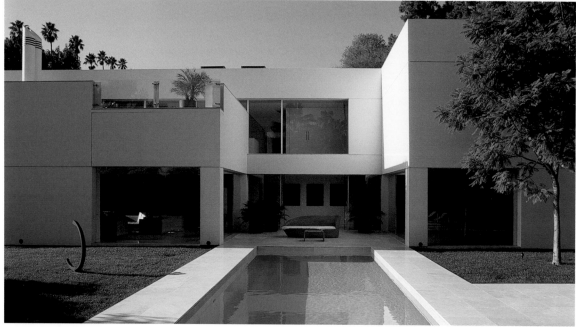

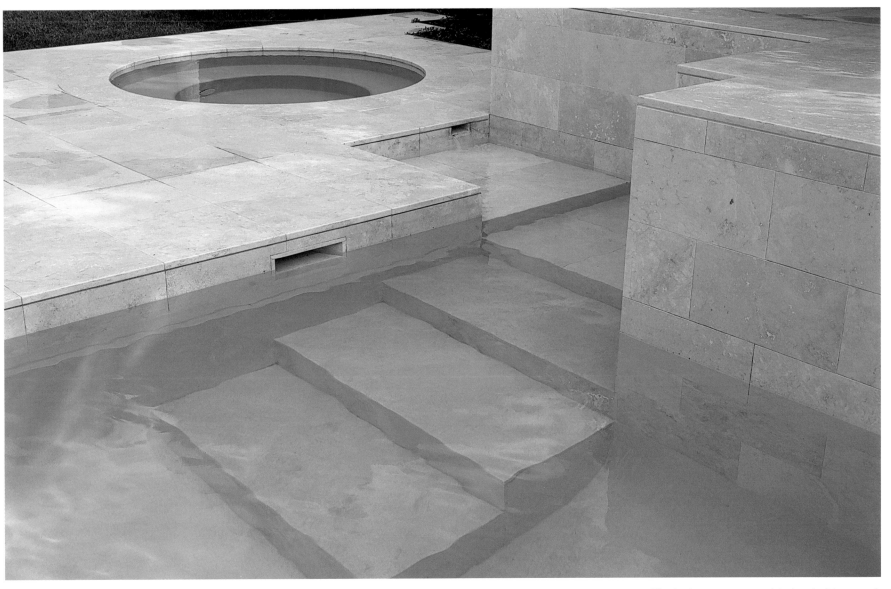

The hydromassage pool is located in a nook surrounded by vegetation, which exudes peace and calm.

Emerson Sauna

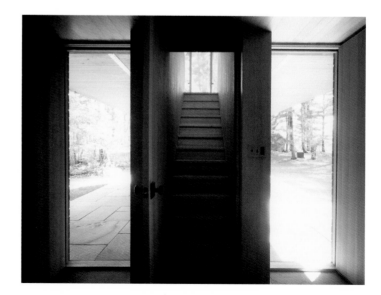

On the farms that Finnish settlers built upon their arrival in the United States, the sauna was often the first building to be built. The clients of this project aimed not just to build another sauna, but to recover the lost social dimension of the practice, which has long since disappeared in other saunas built for private residences. The Emerson Sauna is a large, freestanding building designed to house social gatherings. In the sauna, cooling is as important as heat, and to this end, the sauna was provided with an outdoor shower and a triangular sitting room that would be open to the breeze. The main elements in the sauna are brick and wood, which, in addition to being essential to maintaining heat, help to create a warm and welcoming atmosphere. Oddly enough, despite its technical innovations and the provocative shapes designed by architect David Salmela, the Emerson Sauna is able to evoke the spirit of a traditional sauna.

Architect: **Salmela Architecture and Design**
Location: **Duluth, Minnesota, United States**
Photos © **Peter Bastianelli-Kerze**

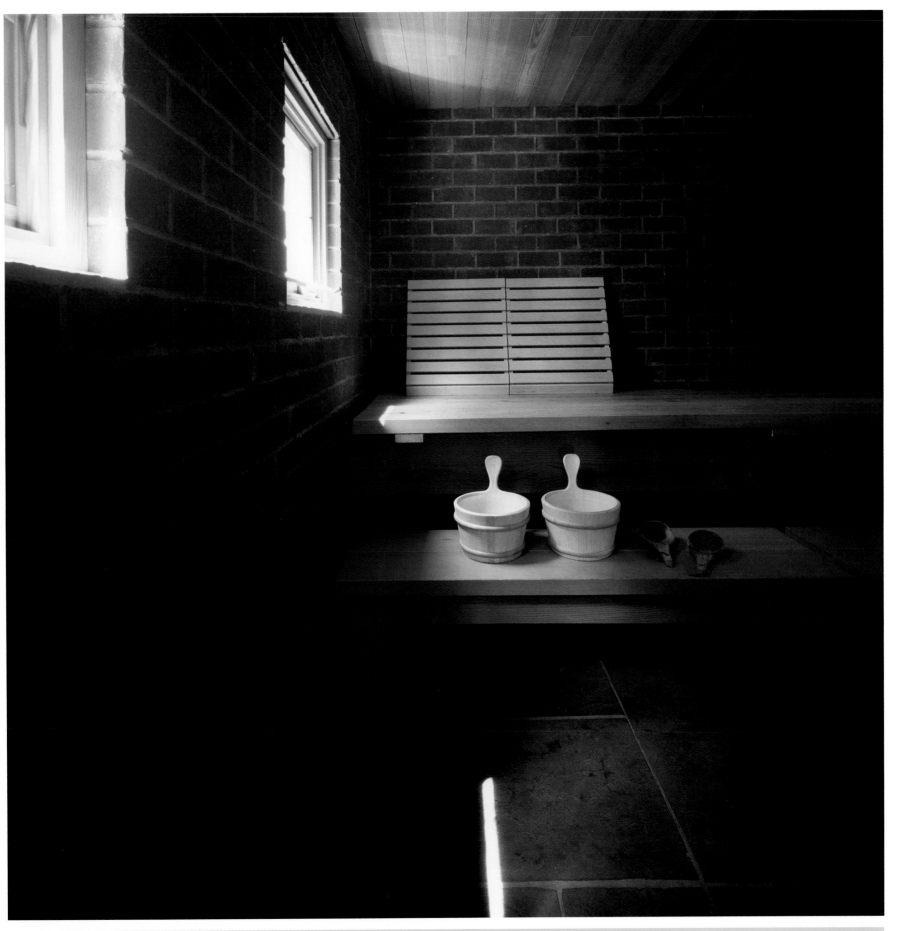

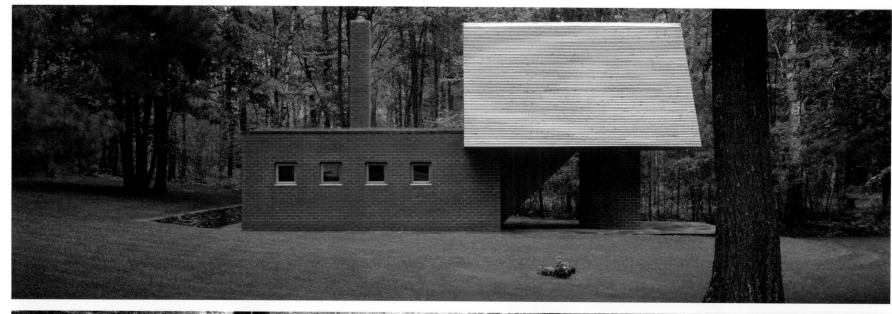

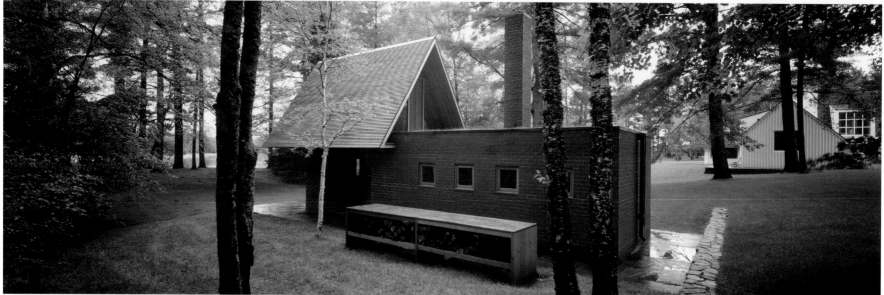

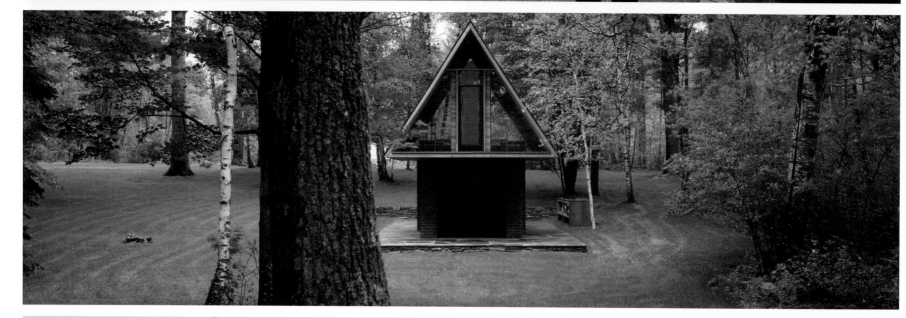

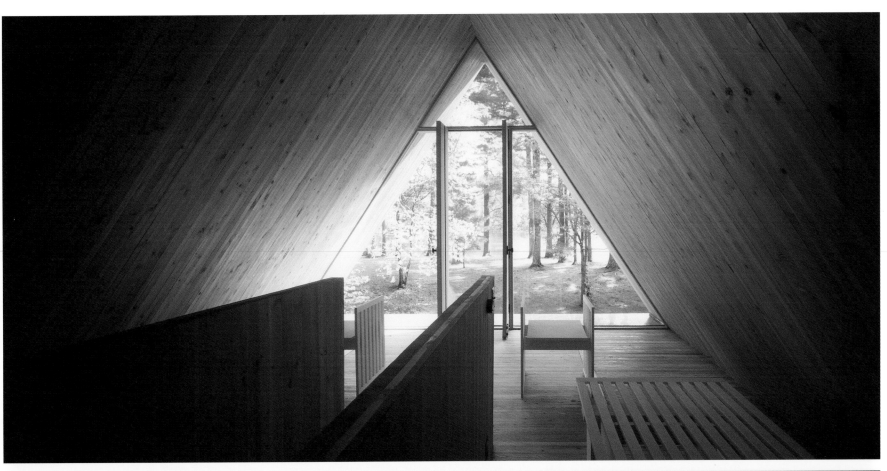

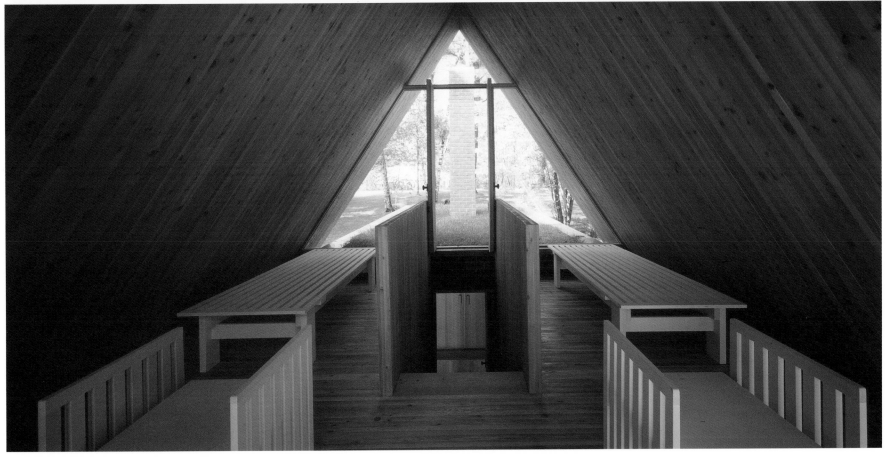

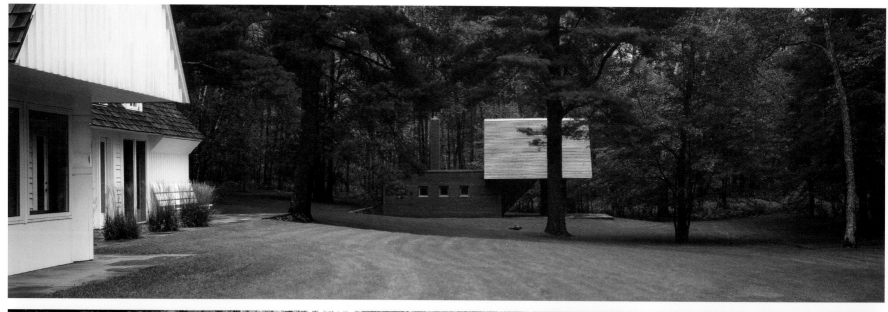

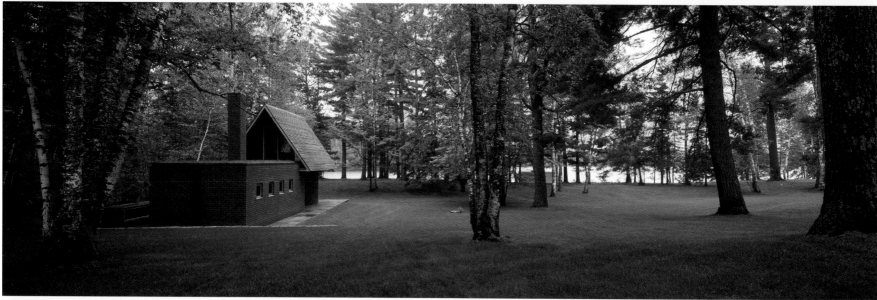

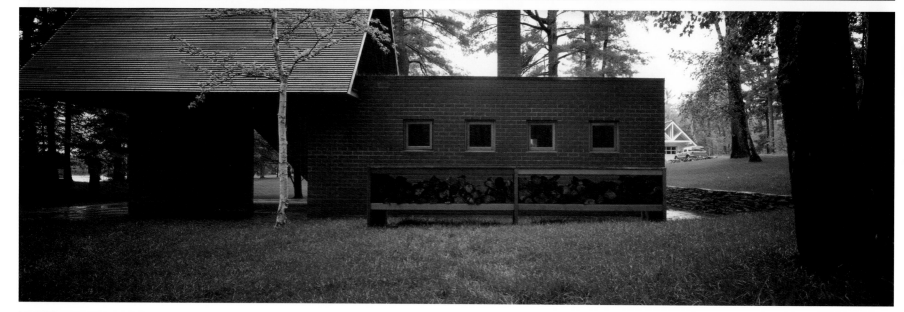

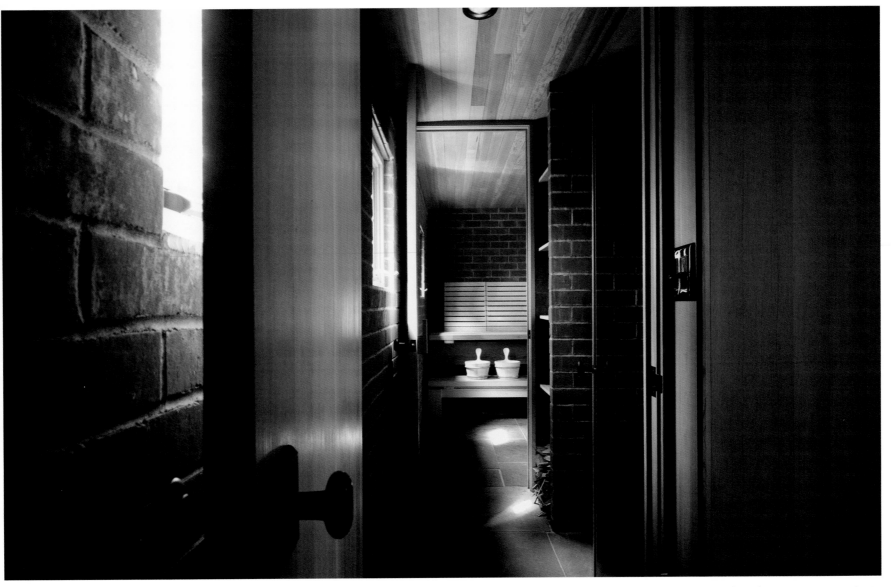

This sauna has the elements one needs to decompress in a unique building dedicated specifically to the purpose.

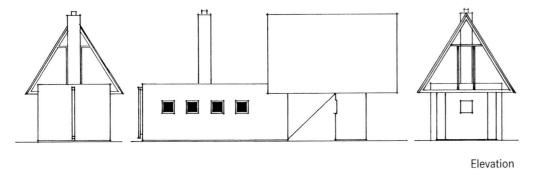

Elevation

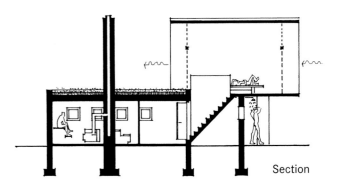

Section

Accessories

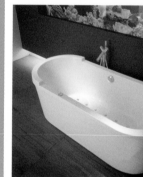

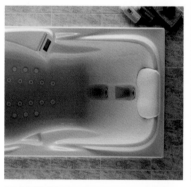

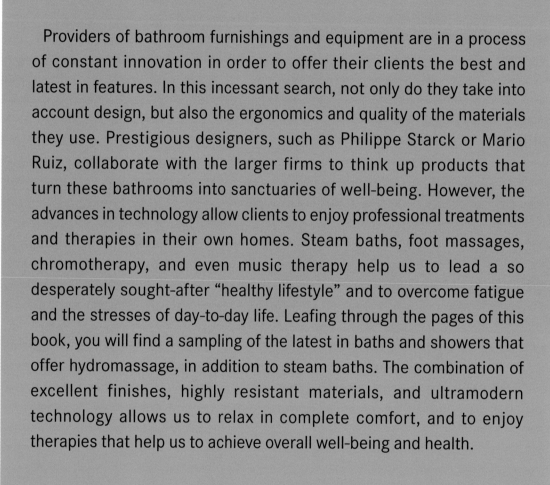

Providers of bathroom furnishings and equipment are in a process of constant innovation in order to offer their clients the best and latest in features. In this incessant search, not only do they take into account design, but also the ergonomics and quality of the materials they use. Prestigious designers, such as Philippe Starck or Mario Ruiz, collaborate with the larger firms to think up products that turn these bathrooms into sanctuaries of well-being. However, the advances in technology allow clients to enjoy professional treatments and therapies in their own homes. Steam baths, foot massages, chromotherapy, and even music therapy help us to lead a so desperately sought-after "healthy lifestyle" and to overcome fatigue and the stresses of day-to-day life. Leafing through the pages of this book, you will find a sampling of the latest in baths and showers that offer hydromassage, in addition to steam baths. The combination of excellent finishes, highly resistant materials, and ultramodern technology allows us to relax in complete comfort, and to enjoy therapies that help us to achieve overall well-being and health.

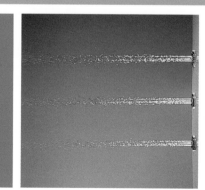

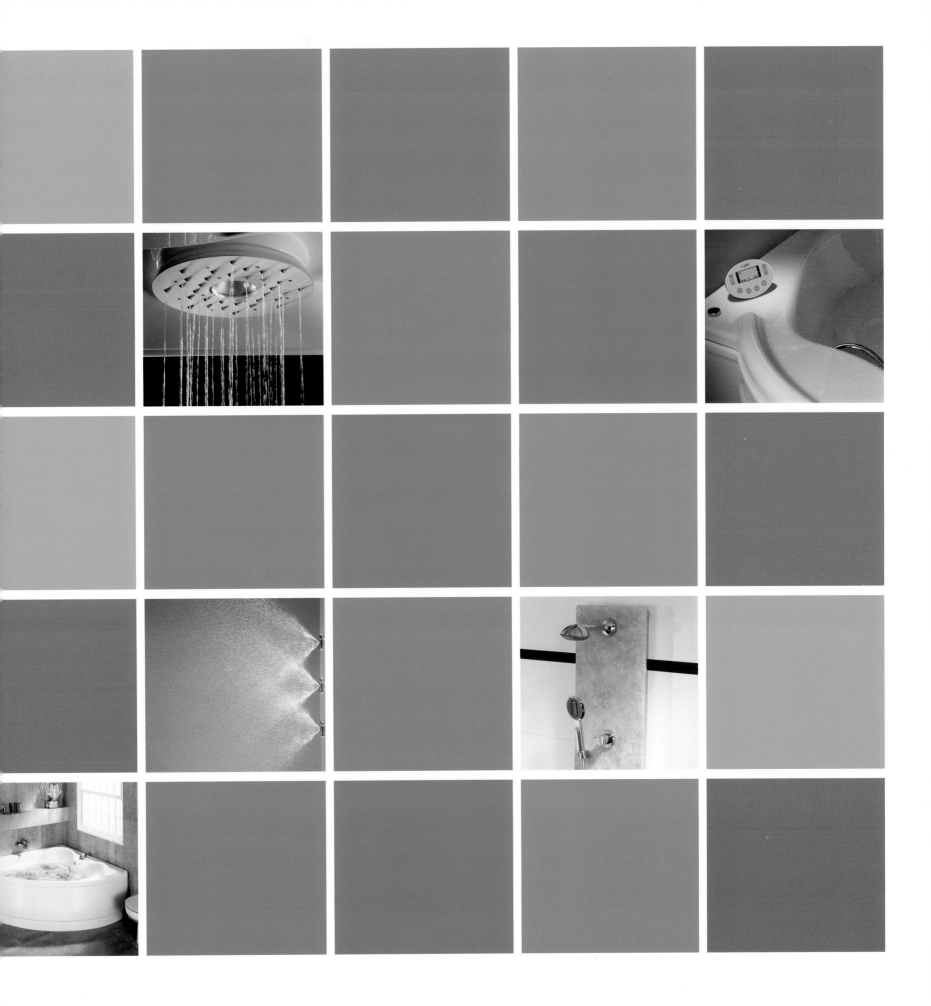

Showers
and Cabins

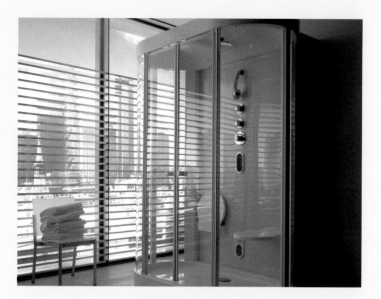

Advances in technology have arrived at the point where one can enjoy the well-being generated by hydromassage showers and cabins in the privacy of one's own home. The companies that manufacture these products have proven themselves able to combine the latest features with exquisitely wrought designs. The result is both practical and functional, as these baths require little space, yet refuse to sacrifice wide ranges of options: in addition to the classic hydromassage, these cabins and columns also offer new systems for lymphatic massage, which is constant and pulsating; the Scottish shower, which incorporates changes in temperature, therapeutic treatments based on ozone, chromotherapy, aromatherapy, foot massage, and steam baths that combine the essences of thyme, eucalyptus, mint, or orange blossoms. Aesthetic trends have yielded a diverse range of materials—encompassing everything from wood to steel—while the design of these baths continues to strive to provide the level of comfort and relaxation needed to enjoy one's home spa to the fullest.

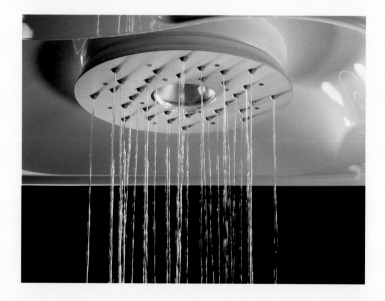

(Top) Steam bath and hydromassage cabin.
Design by Norman Foster for Hoesch.

(Bottom) Ideal Standard cabins' Tropical Rain Effect.

(Next page) Gala's Prisma Block hydromassage column, adaptable to any bath.

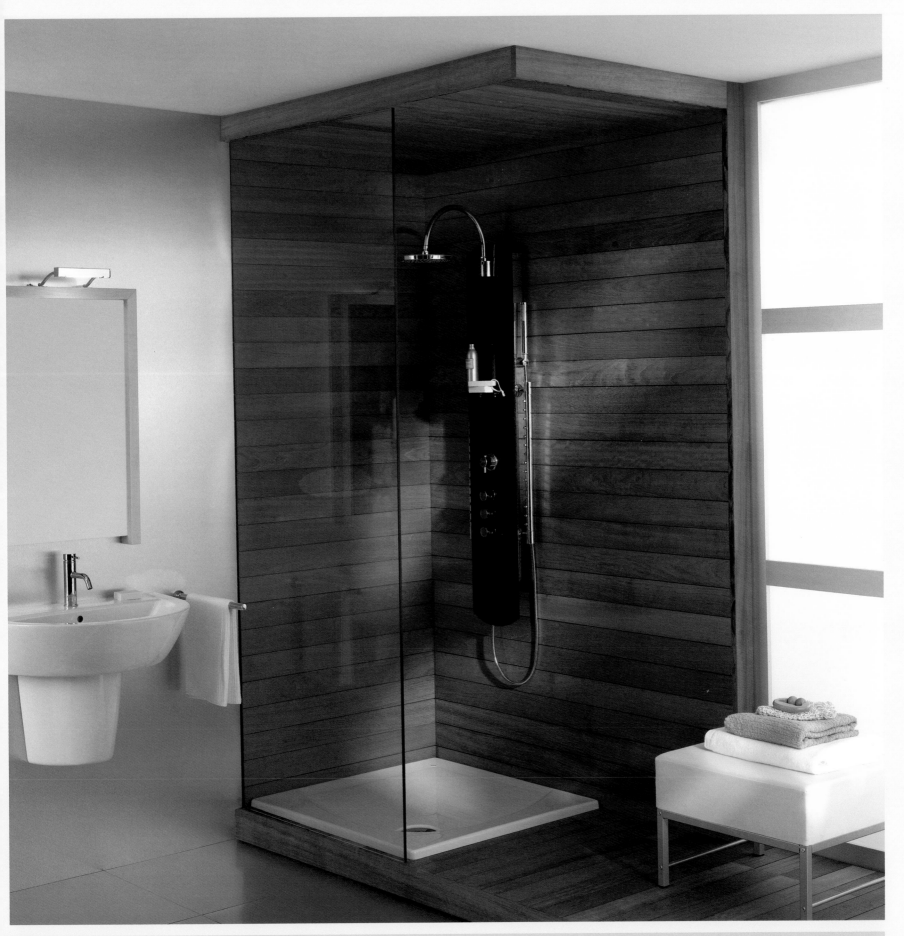

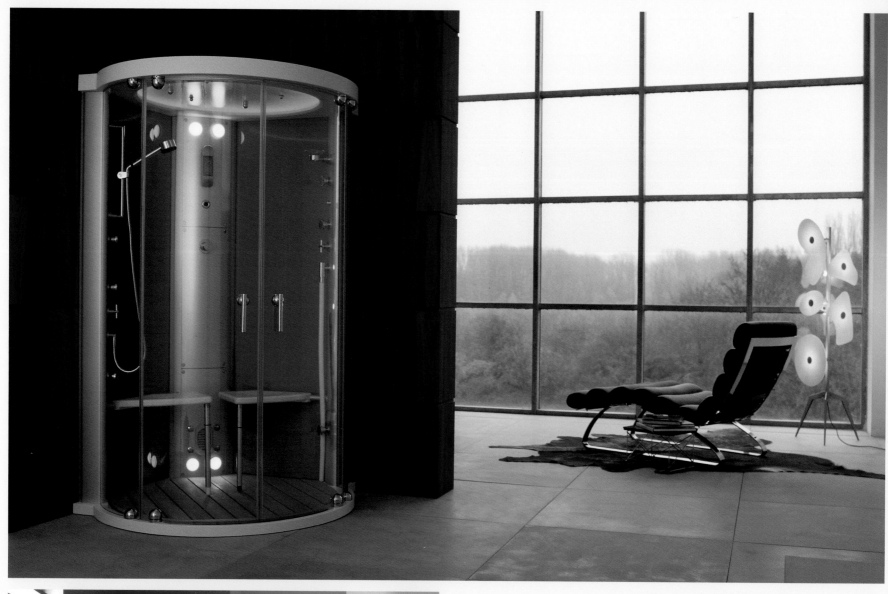

Sensamare 1100 Cabin, designed by Yellow Design/Yellow Circle for Hoesch. Adapted for music, chromotherapy, and aromatherapy.

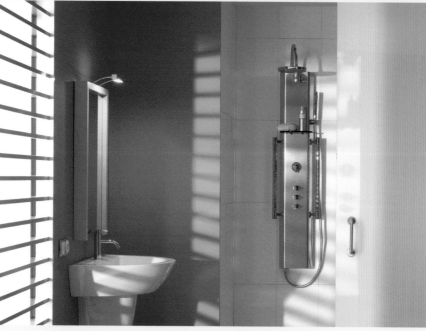

Prisma Inox Column. Its wide range of functions includes thermostatic faucets.

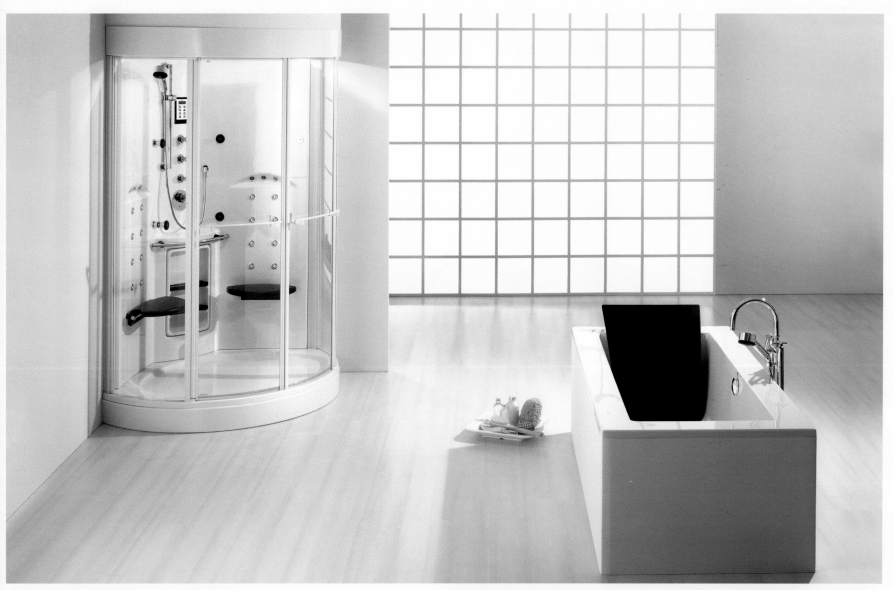

Abano Mini Nova 1100 steam bath and shower, by Hoesch. Seats two people and includes 22 hydromassage jets.

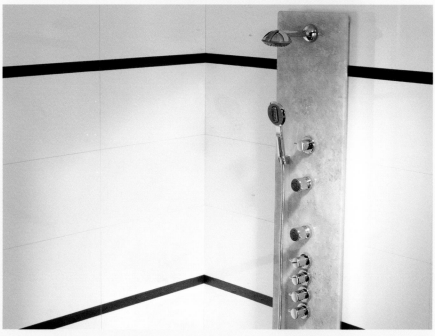

Idea hydromassage column, by Gala. Very easy to install. Includes an air-water massage and thermostatic faucets.

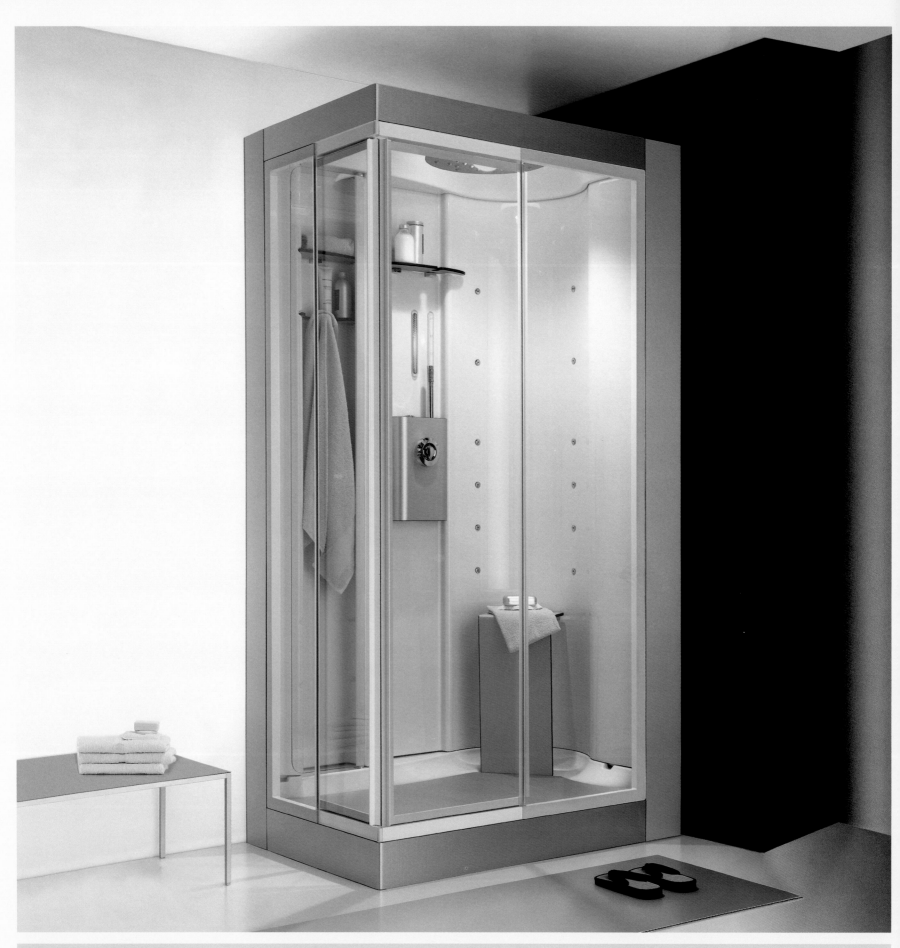

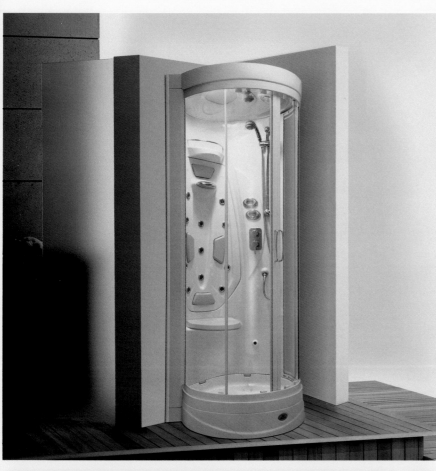

Idea Circular, an individual cabin by Ideal Standard.

(Bottom left) Aquatec cabin, by Roca. It is presented alongside the Zona Paraíso, an auxiliary space in warm wood by Doussie for the utmost in comfort. Of note is the infrared lamp for warming towels.

(Bottom right) Advant cabin, by Roca. Its features define it as a full hydrosauna and include a hydromassage plus steam bath with multifunction jets.

(Previous page) Colorem R steam bath and hydromassage bath, designed by Marc Sadler for Ideal Standard. Of note are its stunning finishes.

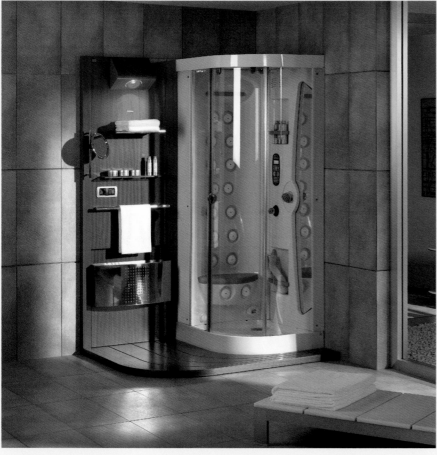

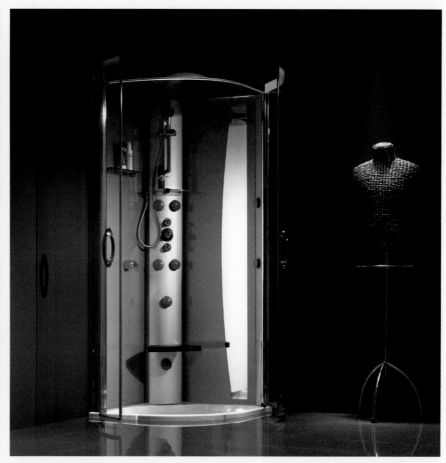

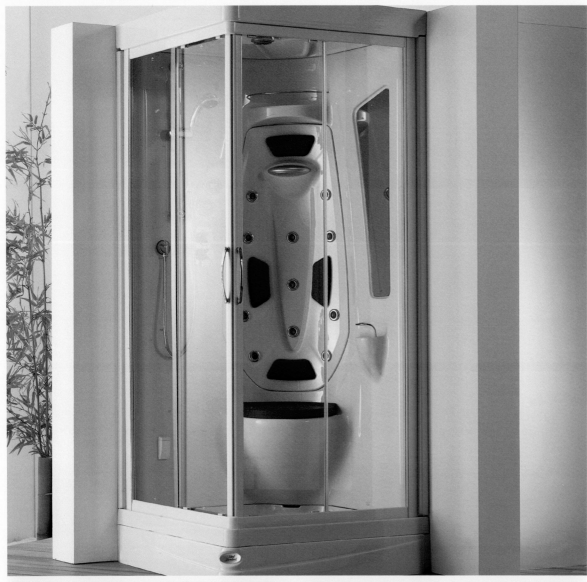

Nereus Idea hydromassage and steam bath, by Ideal Standard. An individual cabin with an extremely comfortable seat.

(Bottom) Ideal Standard cabins' multifunction jets.

(Next page) Arco, by Gala. It includes an electronic panel, chromotherapy, and essential oils, among other features.

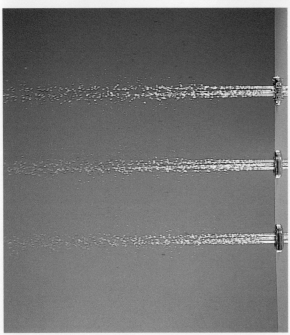

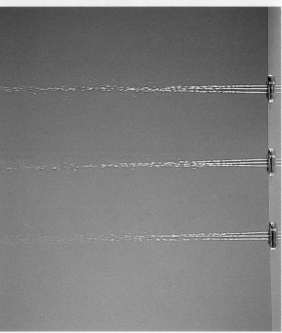

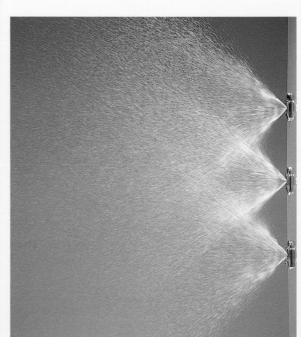

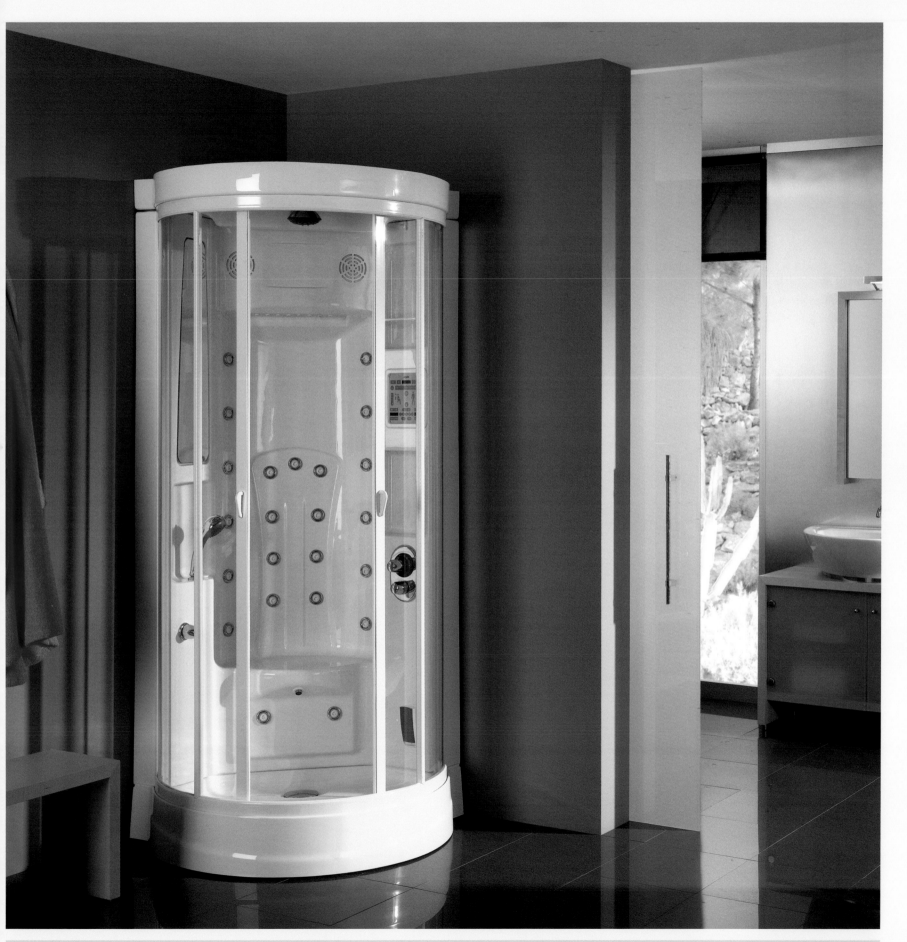

Hydromassage Baths

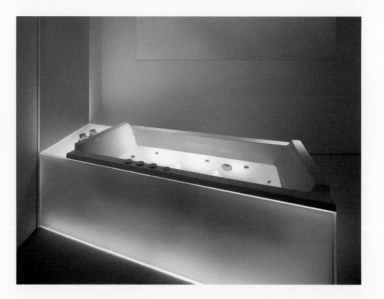

As the role played by the bathroom in the modern home has progressively grown in importance, the choices of hydromassage baths have grown ever larger and more varied to suit. The exhausting rhythm of life to which a substantial part of society is subjected drives the search for new ways of complementing personal hygiene that focus on psychological and physical health, as well as—why not?—on leisure. The current market offers a wide range of hydromassage baths: simple models mix water with air bubbles, others combine water propulsion with air pressure, and even more sophisticated models make use of high-frequency sound waves. Alongside this modernization of hydromassage systems, other features have been added to them, such as chromotherapy or foot massages, to provide users with an experience that is as enjoyable as possible.

(Top)Rectangular bath incorporating chromotherapy, designed by Philippe Starck for Duravit.

(Bottom)Broadway Compact Mini-Pool, by Roca. Adjustable Air-Water Hydromassage and electronic keypad.

(Next page)Kubik Built-In Hydromassage Bath, designed by Mario Ruiz for Bañacril.

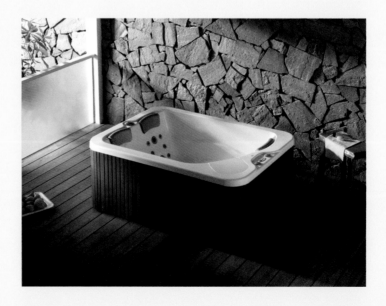

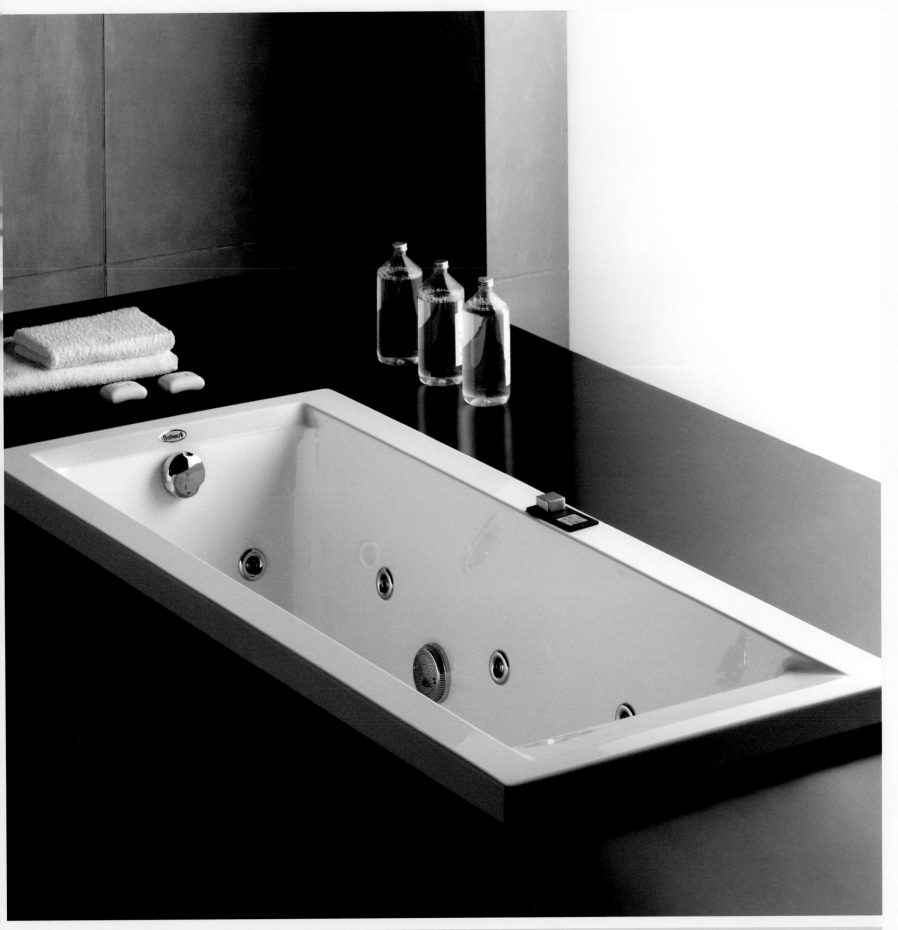

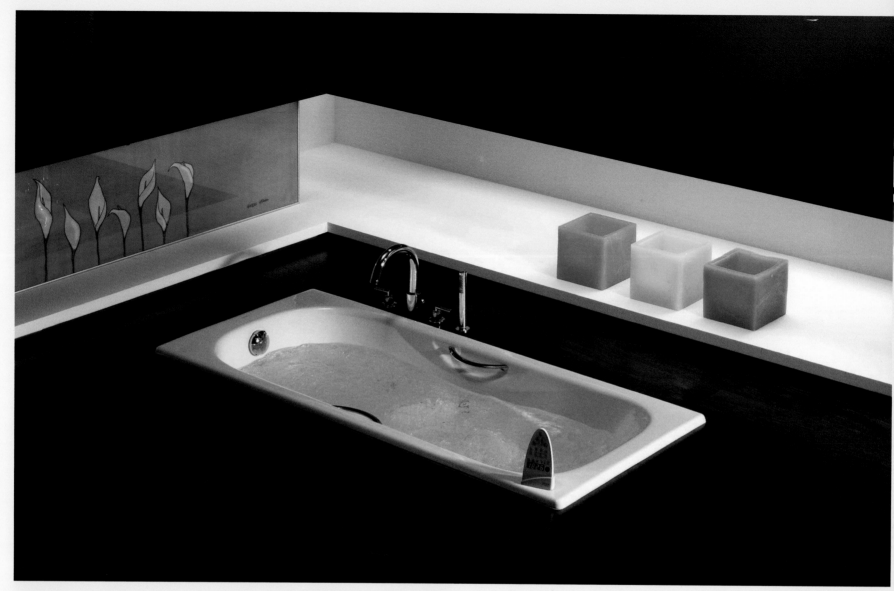

Roca's Malibu model.
Cast-iron tub with air-water massage.

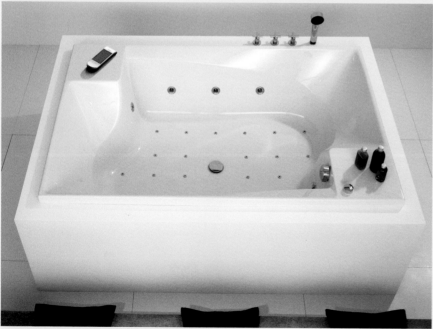

Santee WW Bath, by Adolf Babel for Hoesch.

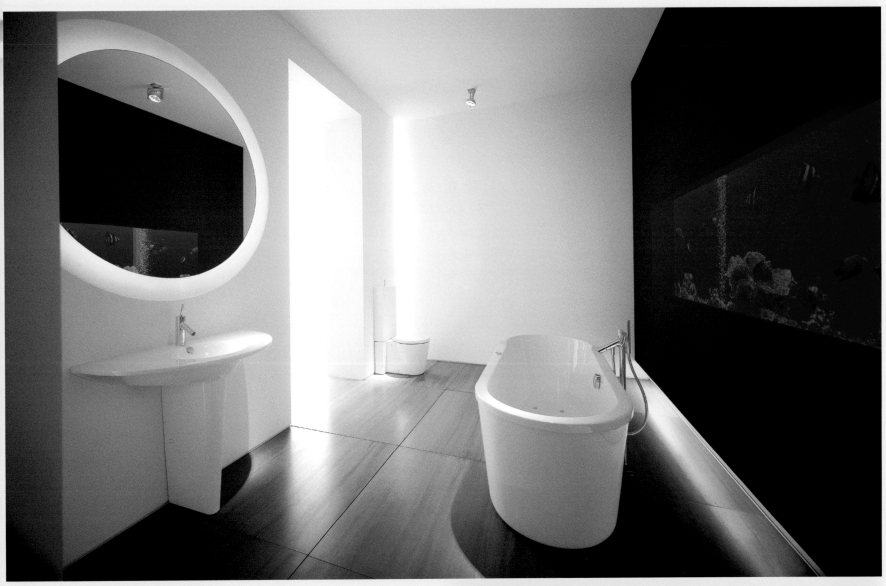

Starck 1 Elegant Bath, by Philippe Starck
for Duravit.

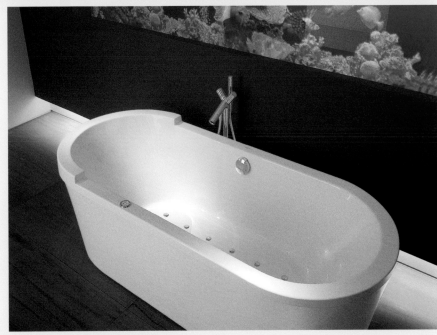

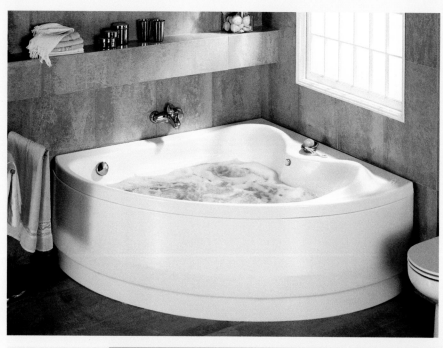

Magia Corner Bath, by Roca.
Includes air-water hydromassage.

Kubik with hydromassage; design by Mario Ruiz
for Bañacril.

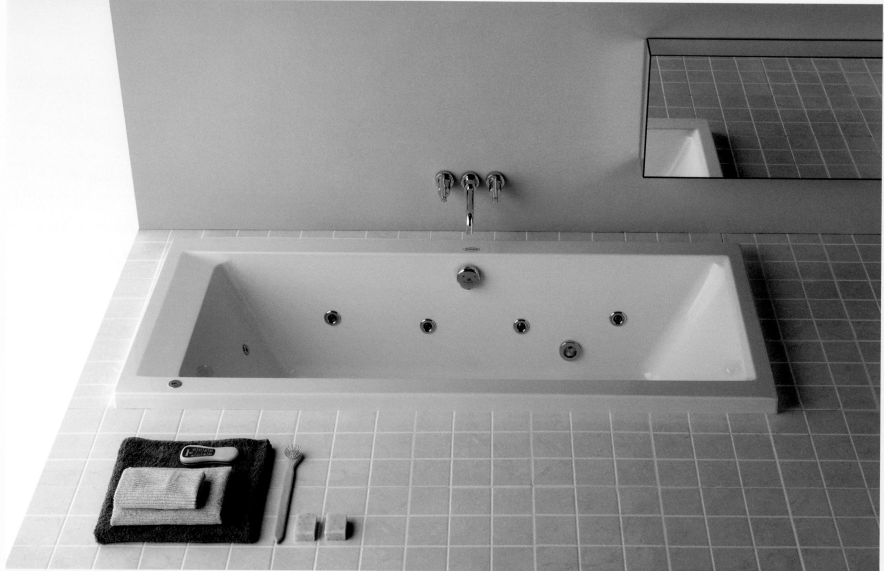

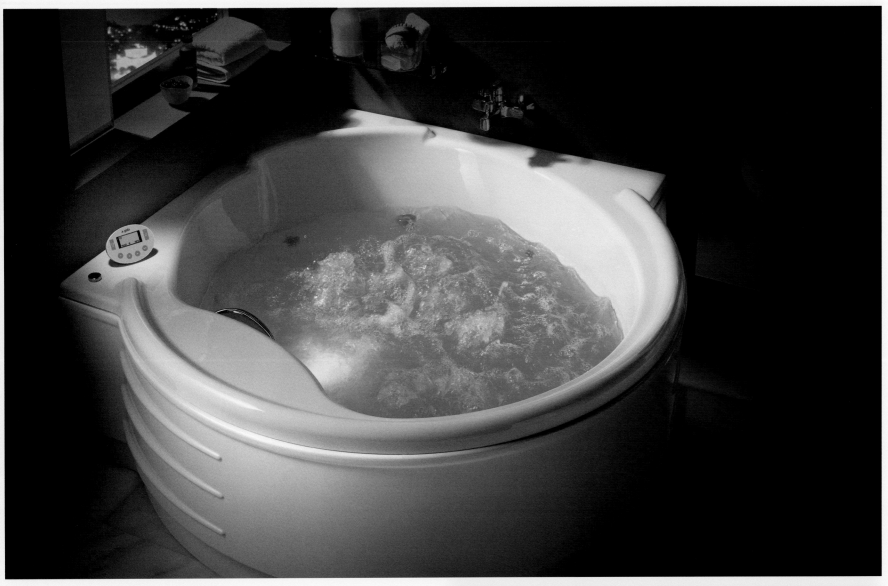

Gala's Estele Air-Water Hydromassage Bath.
A multifunction digital panel is incorporated.

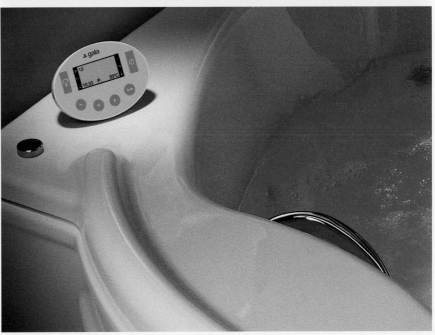

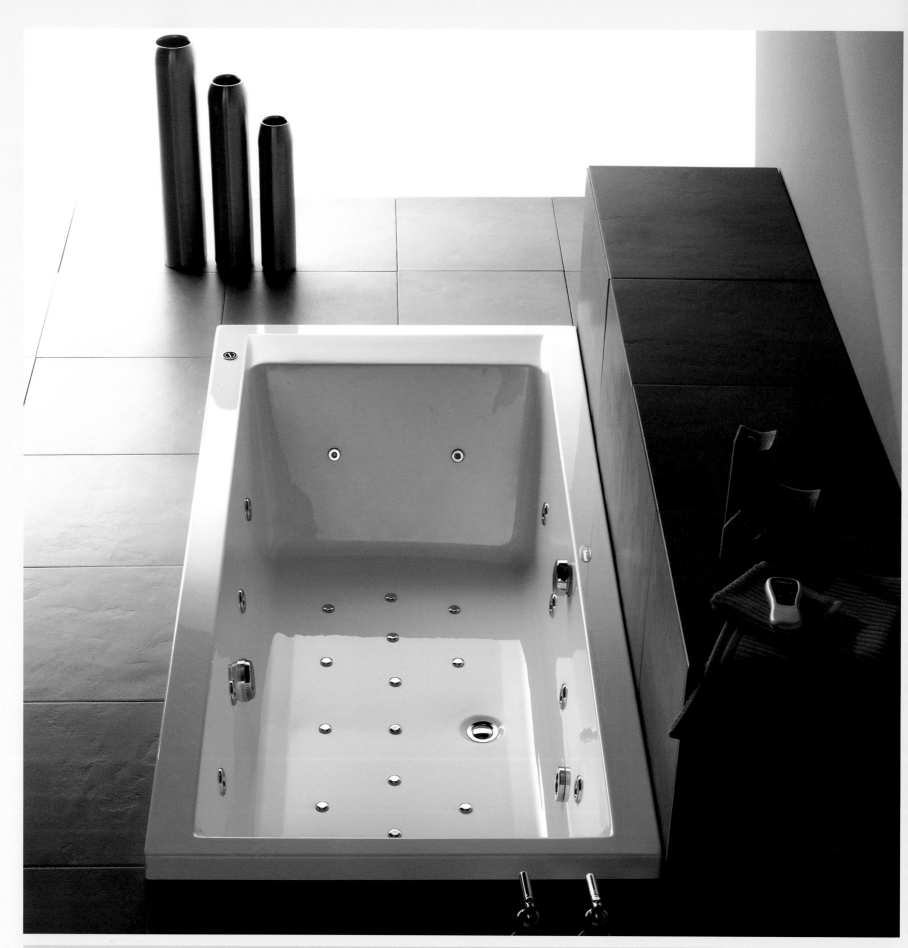

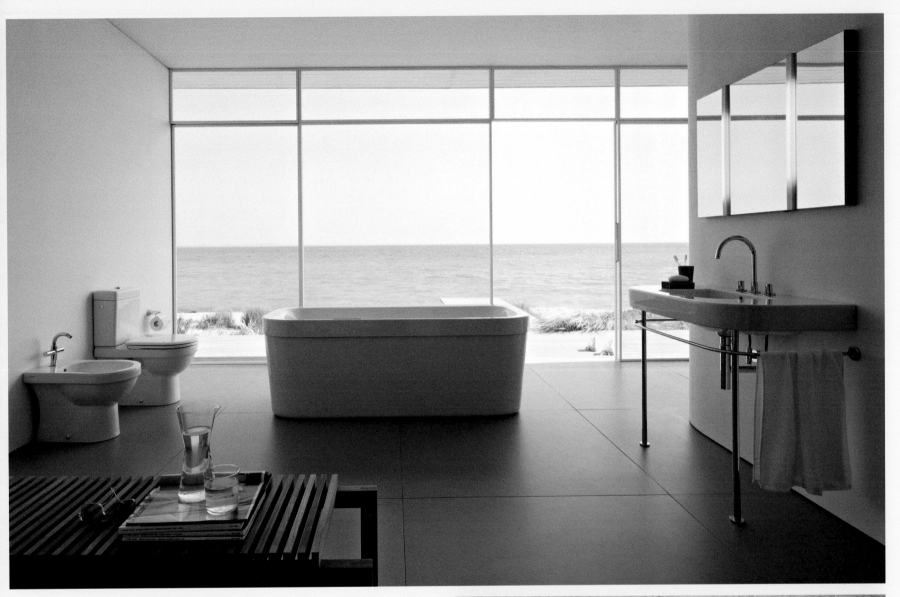

Hydromassage Bath incorporating chromotherapy by Duravit, designed by Sieger Design.

(Previous page) Another model in the elegant Kubik series of hydromassage baths, designed by Mario Ruiz for Bañacril.

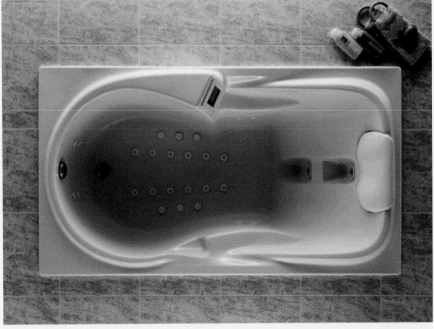

Roca's Karmine model. Programmable, ergonomic, and including a touch screen.

Directory

Anna Generó/Ivalo
Mestre Nicolau, 4
08021 Barcelona, Spain
T./F. + 34 93 200 46 40
M. +34 609 72 57 24

**Anna Popelka, Georg Poduschka/
PPAG Architekten**
Schadekgasse 16/1
1060 Vienna, Austria
T./F. +43 1 587 44 71
po_po@chello.at

Auris Architekten
Steinbergweg 39
64285 Darmstadt, Germany
T. +49(0) 6151 429 7520
F. +49(0) 6151 429 7522
www.aurisgmbh.de
office@aurisgmbh.de

Bárbara Sindreu/Cad Interiorismo
Andana 21, bajos
08190 Sant Cugat del Vallés,
Barcelona, Spain
T. +34 93 674 62 39
M. +34 687 823 827
barbara@cadinteriorismo.com

Bonetti Kozerski Studio
270 Lafayette Street suite 906
New York NY 10012, USA
T. +1 212 343 9898
F. +1 212 343 8042
www.bonettikozerski.com
info@bonettikozerski.com

Candy & Candy
100 Brompton Road, Knightsbridge
London, SW3 1ER
T. +44 (0) 207 594 4300
F. +44 (0) 207 594 4301
www.candyandcandy.com
info@candyandcandy.com

Caña y Caña
Florida 6-8
08120 La Llagosta, Barcelona, Spain

Claesson Koivisto Rune Arkitektkontor
Sankt Paulsgatan 25
118 48 Stockholm, Sweden
T. +46 8 644 58 63
F. +46 8 644 58 83
www.claesson-koivisto-rune.se
arkitektkontor@claesson-koivisto-rune.se

Donald Billinkoff Architects
310 Riverside Drive
Suite 202-1
New York NY 10025, USA
T. +1 212 678 7755
F. +1 212 678 7743
www.billinkoff.com
dba@billinkoff.com

Guilhem Roustan
22 rue de la Folie Méricourt
75011 Paris, France
T. +33 01 43 55 80 04
F. +33 01 40 21 69 14
www.roustanarchitecture.com
gr@roustanarchitecture.com

Jaime Sanahuja
Fernando el Católico 34, bajos
12005 Castellón, Spain
T. +34 964 724 949
www.jaimesanahuja.com

Jones Studio
4450 N. 12th St. Suite 104
AZ 85014 Phoenix, USA
T. +1 602 264 2941
F. +1 602 264 3440
www.jonesstudioinc.com

Jorge Segarra
M. +34 607 231 705
09039@ctav.es

Legorreta y Legorreta
Palacio de Versalles 285-A
Mexico DF 11020, Mexico
T. +52 55 5251 9698
F. +52 55 5596 6162
legorret@lmasl.com.mx

Leopoldo Rosati
300 East 40th Street
10s New York NY 10016, USA
T. +1 212 983 0929
F. +1 212 983 0933
www.leopoldorosati.com
leoros@mac.com

Lilia Konrad/LKD Concepts
Neuhausstrasse 3
6318 Zug, Switzerland
T./F. +41 41 758 22 49

Marcio Kogan
Al. Tietê, 505, São Paulo
Cep 04616-001 Brazil
T. +55 11 308 135 22
F. +55 11 306 334 24
www.marciokogan.com.br
mk-mk@uol.com.br

Marmol Radziner and Associates
12210 Nebraska Avenue
Los Angeles, CA 90025, USA
T. +1 310 826 6222
F. +1 310 826 6226
www.marmol-radziner.com

Mikael Bergquist Arkitektkontor
Kvarngatan 14
118 47 Stockholm, Sweden
T. +46 08 765 72 35
F. +46 08 702 15 45
www.mba.nu
mb@mba.nu

Moiseś Becker
Becker Arquitectos
Monte Libano 235 P.B.
Mexico 11000, D.F., Mexico

Olle Lundberg/Lundberg Design
2620 Third Street
San Francisco, CA 94107, USA
T. +1 415 695 0110 18
F. +1 415 695 0379
www.lundbergdesign.com

Raquel Chamorro/Quattrocento
General Díaz Porlier 51
28001 Madrid, Spain
T. +34 91 309 67 04
F. +34 91 402 49 35
M. +34 610 438 644 - +34 650 717 662
www.raquelchamorro.com
correo@raquelchamorro.com

Salmela Architecture and Design
852 Grandview Avenue
55812 Duluth, Minnesota, USA
T. +1 218 724 7517
F. +1 218 728 6805
ddsalmela@charter.net

Samuel Lerch
Eibenstr. 9
8045 Zurich, Switzerland
T. +41 1 382 4655
samnad@swissonline.ch

Satoshi Okada Architects
16-12-302/303 Tomihisa, Shinjuku
Tokyo 162-0067, Japan
T. +81 3 3355 0646
F. +81 3 3355 0658
www.satoshi-archi.com
satoshi@okada-archi.com

Studiomonti
Piazza Sant'Erasmo 1,
20121 Milan, Italy
T. +39 02 6599470
F. +39 02 29019795
www.studiomonti.com
info@studiomonti.com

Studio Rinaldi
250 W 57th ST#1210
New York, NY 10107, USA
T. +1 212 581 2314
F. +1 212 581 2524
www.studiosrinaldi.com
srinaldi@studiosrinaldi.com

Studio Salizzoni
Via del Riccio 4
40123 Bologna, Italy
T. +39 051 33 11 37
F. +39 051 58 24 65
gsalizzo@tin.it

**Takaharu + Yiu Tezuka/Tezuka Architects,
Masahiro Ikeda/mias**
1-19-9-3F Todoroki Setagaya
158-0082 – Tokyo, Japan
T. +81 03-3703-7056
F. +81 03-3703-7038
www.tezuka-arch.com
tez@sepia.ocn.ne.jp

Ulf Norr/MFA Kupé Corporation
Häggtunet 18
181 48 Lidingö, Stockholm, Sweden
T. +46 708 929 956
www.kupe.se
ulf.norr@kupe.se

Ignacio Vicens and José Antonio Ramos
Barquillo 29, 2º izq.
28004 Madrid, Spain
T. +34 91 521 0004
F. +34 91 521 6550
vicensramos@arquired.es

Wingårdh
Kungsgatan 10A
411 19 Göteborg, Sweden
T. + 46 (0) 31 743 70 00
F. +46 (0) 31 711 98 38
www.wingardhs.se
wingardhs@wingardhs.se

Spas for Your Home—Sources

Agape Design
P.O. Box 1668
New York, NY 10013
Phone: 1-212-941-9941
Web: www.agapedesign.it
E-mail: info@agapedesign.it

Amerec Sauna and Steam
17683 128th Place NE, #C
Woodinville, WA 98072
Phone: 1-425-951-1120
Toll-Free: 1-800-331-0349
Fax: 1-425-951-1130
Web: www.amerec.com
E-mail: amerec@earthlink.net

American Jetted Bathtubs
1622 North Magnolia Avenue
El Cajon, CA 92020
Toll-Free: 1-800-817-1977
Fax: 1-619-596-2431
Web: www.americanjettedbathtubs.com
E-mail: info@americanjettedbathtubs.com

American Standard
P.O. Box 6820
1 Centennial Plaza
Piscataway, NJ 08855-6820
Phone: 1-612-375-8516
Toll-Free: 1-800-442-1902
Web: www.americanstandard-us.com

Americh Corp.
(East Coast)
10700 John Price Road
Charlotte, NC 28273
Phone: 1-704-588-3075
Fax: 1-704-588-3166
(West Coast)
13212 Saticoy Street
North Hollywood, CA 91605
Phone: 1-818-982-1711
Fax: 1-818-982-2764
Web: www.americh.com

Aqua Glass Corporation
320 Industrial Park Drive
Adamsville, TN 38310
Phone: 1-731-632-2501
Toll-Free: 1-800-435-7875
Fax: 1-800-822-9011
Web: www.aquaglass.com

Aquarius Bathware
435 Industrial Road
Savannah, TN 38372
Phone: 1-731-925-7656
Toll-Free: 1-800-443-7269
Fax: 1-731-925-0379
Web: www.aquariusproducts.com

Aroma Spas
A Division of Rosebud Industries, Inc.
1622 North Magnolia Avenue
El Cajon, CA 92020
Phone: 1-619-596-6435
Toll-Free: 1-800-927-6110
Fax: 1-619-596-6439
Web: www.aromaspas.com
E-mail: info@aromaspas.com

Bañacril
Torres Quevedo, s/n
Pol. Ind. Coll de la Manya
08400 Granollers, Spain
Phone: 011-34-93-860-88-00
Fax: 011-34-93-860-88-04
Web: www.banacril.com

Cabuchon Bathforms
Whitegate, Lancaster
LA3 3BT
United Kingdom
Phone: 011-44-01524-66022
Fax: 011-44-01524-844927
Web: www.cabuchon.com
E-mail: info@cabuchon.com

Convectair NMT Inc.
30 Carré Sicard
Sainte-Thérèse, Quebec
J7E 3X6 Canada
Phone: 1-450-433-5701
Toll-Free: 1-800-463-6478
Fax: 1-450-433-5701
Web: www.convectair.com

Davis & Warshow
57-22 49th Street
Maspeth, NY 11378
Phone: 1-718-937-9500
Fax: 1-718-786-7711
Web: www.daviswarshow.com
E-mail: info@davidwarshow.com

Duravit USA
1750 Breckinridge Parkway, Suite 500
Duluth, GA 30096
Phone: 1-770-931-3575
Toll-Free: 1-888-387-2848
Fax: 1-770-931-8454
Web: www.duravit.us
E-mail: info@usa.duravit.com

Endless Pools
200 East Dutton Mill Road
Aston, PA 19014
Phone: 1-610-497-8676
Toll-Free: 1-800-732-8660
Web: www.endlesspools.com

Floataway
14-17 Ironside Way
Hingham, Norfolk
NR9 4LF
United Kingdom
Phone: 011-44-1953-85-15-15
Fax: 011-44-1953-851-861
Web: www.floataway.com

Finnleo Sauna and Steam
575 East Cokato Street
Cokato, MN 55321
Phone: 1-320-286-5584
Toll-Free: 1-800-346-6536
Fax: 1-320-286-6100
Web: www.finnleo.com
E-mail: finnleo@saunatec.com

Gala
Ctra. de Madrid
Irún, Km. 244
Apdo. 293
09080 Burgos
Spain
Phone: 011-34-947-47-41-00
Fax: 011-34-947-47-41-03
Web: www.gala.es
E-mail: general@gala.es

Health Essentials
4607 Lakeview Canyon #101
Westlake Village, CA 91361
Phone: 1-818-706-1888
Toll-Free: 1-800-653-8881
Web: www.healthessentials4you.com

Helo Sauno and Steam
575 East Cokato Street
Cokato, MN 55321
Phone: 1-320-286-6304
Toll-Free: 1-800-882-4352
Fax: 1-320-286-2224
Web: www.helosaunas.com
E-mail: helo@saunatec.com

Hoesch America Inc.
2805 Veterans Highway, Suite 7
Ronkonkoma, NY 11779
Phone: 1-631-737-3797
Fax: 1-631-737-4037
Web: www.hoesch.de
E-mail: info@hoeschamerica.com